THE AIDS CRISIS

Conflicting Social Values

Gary E. McCuen

IDEAS IN CONFLICT SERIES

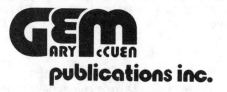
GEM
GARY McCUEN
publications inc.

411 Mallalieu Drive
Hudson, Wisconsin 54016
phone (715) 386-5662

Illustration & photo credits
Chuck Asay 124, Jerry Fearing 141, Jack Hamm 82, 93, Craig Macintosh
39, 43, 50, *The Militant* 73, Eleanor Mill 21, 108, Pat Mitchell 60,
Oliphant 88, Bill Sanders 132, 145, David Seavey 13, 26, 115.

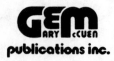

© 1987 by Gary E. McCuen Publications, Inc.
411 Mallalieu Drive • Hudson, Wisconsin 54016
 (715) 386-5662
publications inc. International Standard Book Number 0-86596-061-5
Printed in the United States of America

CONTENTS

CHAPTER 4   THE POLITICS OF AIDS

REASONING SKILL DEVELOPMENT

These activities may be used as individualized study guides for students in libraries and resource centers or as discussion catalysts in small group and classroom discussions.

IDEAS in CONFLICT ®

This series features ideas in conflict on political, social and moral issues. It presents counterpoints, debates, opinions, commentary and analysis for use in libraries and classrooms. Each title in the series uses one or more of the following basic elements:

Introductions that present an issue overview giving historic background and/or a description of the controversy.

Counterpoints and debates carefully chosen from publications, books, and position papers on the political right and left to help librarians and teachers respond to requests that treatment of public issues be fair and balanced.

Symposiums and forums that go beyond debates that can polarize and oversimplify. These present commentary from across the political spectrum that reflect how complex issues attract many shades of opinion.

*A **global** emphasis with foreign perspectives and surveys on various moral questions and political issues that will help readers to place subject matter in a less culture-bound and ethno-centric frame of reference. In an ever shrinking and interdependent world, understanding and cooperation are essential. Many issues are global in nature and can be effectively dealt with only by common efforts and international understanding.*

Reasoning skill study guides and discussion activities provide ready made tools for helping with critical reading and evaluation of content. The guides and activities deal with one or more of the following:

RECOGNIZING AUTHOR'S POINT OF VIEW

INTERPRETING EDITORIAL CARTOONS

VALUES IN CONFLICT

WHAT IS EDITORIAL BIAS?

WHAT IS SEX BIAS?
WHAT IS POLITICAL BIAS?
WHAT IS ETHNOCENTRIC BIAS?
WHAT IS RACE BIAS?
WHAT IS RELIGIOUS BIAS?

*From across **the political spectrum** varied sources are presented for research projects and classroom discussions. Diverse opinions in the series come from magazines, newspapers, syndicated columnists, books, political speeches, foreign nations, and position papers by corporations and non-profit institutions.*

About the Editor

Gary E. McCuen is an editor and publisher of anthologies for public libraries and curriculum materials for schools. Over the past 16 years his publications of over 200 titles have specialized in social, moral and political conflict. They include books, pamphlets, cassettes, tabloids, filmstrips and simulation games, many of them designed from his curriculums during 11 years of teaching junior and senior high school social studies. At present he is the editor and publisher of the *Ideas in Conflict* series and the *Editorial Forum* series.

CHAPTER 1

OVERVIEW

OVERVIEW

FACTS ABOUT AIDS

Public Health Service

The Acquired Immune Deficiency Syndrome, or AIDS, was first reported in the United States in mid-1981. Since that time, the Public Health Service has received reports of more than 15,000 cases, about 52 percent of which have resulted in death. An estimated 500,000 to 1 million people have been infected by the virus that causes AIDS, but have no symptoms of illness.

AIDS is a public health problem that merits serious concern. It has been named the number one priority of the U.S. Public Health Service. Researchers in the Public Health Service and in many major medical institutions have been working for more than four years to study AIDS and develop treatments and preventive measures.

This fact sheet describes, in question-and-answer form, accurate information about AIDS, the risk of contracting AIDS, the actions individuals can take to reduce spreading AIDS, and current research and related activities under way in the Public Health Service.

What is AIDS?

AIDS is characterized by a defect in natural immunity against disease. People who have AIDS are vulnerable to serious illnesses which would not be a threat to anyone whose immune system was functioning normally. These illnesses are referred to as "opportunistic" infections or diseases.

Reprinted from *Facts About AIDS* by the U.S. Department of Health and Human Services, Winter, 1986.

What causes AIDS?

Investigators have discovered the virus that causes AIDS. Different groups of investigators have given different names to the virus, but they all appear to be the same virus. The virus is called human T-lymphotropic virus, type III (HTLV-III); lymphadenopathy-associated virus (LAV); or AIDS-related virus (ARV). Infection with this virus does not always lead to AIDS. Preliminary results of studies show that most infected persons remain in good health; others may develop illness varying in severity from mild to extremely serious.

How is AIDS transmitted?

AIDS is spread by sexual contact, needle sharing, or less commonly, through transfused blood or its components. The risk of infection with the virus is increased by having multiple sexual partners, either homosexual or heterosexual, and sharing needles among those using illicit drugs. The occurrence of the syndrome in hemophilia patients and persons receiving transfusions provides evidence for transmission through blood. It may be transmitted from infected mother to infant before, during, or shortly after birth (probably through breast milk).

Who gets AIDS?

Ninety-five percent of the AIDS cases have occurred in the following groups of people:
- Sexually active homosexual and bisexual men, 73 percent;
- Present or past abusers of intravenous drugs, 17 percent;*
- Persons with hemophilia or other coagulation disorders, 1 percent;
- Heterosexual contacts of someone with AIDS or at risk for AIDS, 1 percent;
- Persons who have had transfusions with blood or blood products, 2 percent;
- Infants born to infected mothers, 1 percent.

Some 5% of patients do not fall into any of these groups, but researchers believe that transmission occurred in similar ways. Some patients died before complete histories could be

* In addition, a certain number of homosexual or bisexual men are also I.V. drug users.

taken. Infants and children who have developed AIDS may have been exposed to HTLV-III before or during birth, or shortly thereafter, or may have received transfusions.

What are its Symptoms?

Most individuals infected with the AIDS virus have no symptoms and feel well. Some develop symptoms which may include tiredness, fever, loss of appetite and weight, diarrhea, night sweats, and swollen glands (lymph nodes)—usually in the neck, armpits, or groin. Anyone with these symptoms which continue for more than two weeks should see a doctor.

How long after infection with HTLV-III does a person develop AIDS?

The time between infection with the HTLV-III virus and the onset of symptoms (the incubation period) seems to range from about 6 months to 5 years and possibly longer. Not everyone exposed to the virus develops AIDS.

How is AIDS diagnosed?

There are no clear-cut symptoms that indicate the loss of immunity. The diagnosis of AIDS depends on the presence of opportunistic diseases. Certain tests which demonstrate damage to various parts of the immune system, such as specific types of white blood cells, support the diagnosis. The presence of opportunistic diseases plus a positive test for antibodies to HTLV-III can also make possible a diagnosis of AIDS.

What is the geographic distribution of reported AIDS cases?

Thirty-five percent of the cases in the U.S. are reported from New York State and about 23 percent from California. AIDS cases have been reported from all 50 states, the District of Columbia, Puerto Rico, and more than 35 other countries.

How contagious is AIDS?

Casual contact with AIDS patients or persons who might be at risk for the illness does *not* place others at risk for getting the illness. No cases have been found where the virus has been transmitted by casual household contact with AIDS patients or persons at higher risk for getting the illness. Infants with AIDS or HTLV-III infection have not transmitted the infection to family members living in the same household.

Although the AIDS virus has been found in saliva and tears, there have been no cases in which exposure to either was shown to result in transmission. Ambulance drivers, police, and firefighters who have assisted AIDS patients have not become ill. Nurses, doctors, and health care personnel have not developed AIDS from caring for AIDS patients. Two health care workers in the U.S. have developed antibodies to HTLV-III following needlestick injuries.

Health care and laboratory workers should follow standard safety procedures carefully when handling any blood and tissue samples from patients with potentially transmissible diseases, including AIDS. Special care should be taken to avoid needlestick injuries.

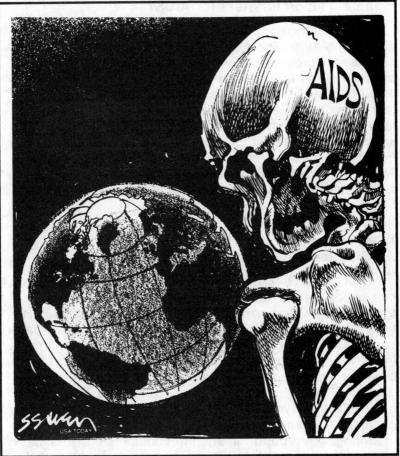

By David Seavey, USA TODAY

Is there a danger of contracting AIDS from donating blood?

No. Blood banks and other blood collection centers use sterile equipment and disposable needles. The need for blood is always acute, and people who are not at increased risk for getting AIDS are urged to continue to donate blood as they have in the past.

Is there a laboratory test for AIDS?

As with many other diseases, there is no single test for diagnosing AIDS. There is now a test for antibodies (substances produced in the blood to fight disease organisms) to the virus that causes AIDS. Presence of HTLV-III antibodies means that a person has been infected with that virus; it does not tell whether the person is still infected. The antibody test is used to screen donated blood and plasma and assist in preventing cases of AIDS resulting from blood transfusions or use of blood products, such as Factor VIII, needed by patients with hemophilia. The test is also available through private physicians, most State or local health departments and at other sites.

What are some of the diseases affecting AIDS patients?

About 82 percent of the AIDS patients studied have had one or both of two rare diseases: *Pneumocystis carinii* pneumonia (PCP), a parasitic infection of the lungs; and a type of cancer known as Kaposi's sarcoma (KS). KS usually occurs anywhere on the surface of the skin or in the mouth. In early stages, it may look like a bruise or blue-violet or brownish spot. The spot or spots persist, and may grow larger. KS may spread to, or appear in, other organs of the body. PCP has symptoms similar to any other form of severe pneumonia, especially cough, fever, and difficulty in breathing. Other opportunistic infections include unusually severe infections with yeast, cytomegalovirus, herpesvirus, and parasites such as *Toxoplasma* or *Cryptosporidia.* Milder infections with these organisms do not suggest immune deficiency.

Is there a danger of a child's contracting AIDS from friends or schoolmates?

No. AIDS is difficult to catch, even among people at highest risk for the disease. The risk of transmitting AIDS from daily contact at work, school, or at home apparently is nonexistent. In virtually all cases, direct sexual contact or the sharing of IV (intravenous) drug needles has led to the illness.

How is AIDS treated?

Currently, there are no antiviral drugs available anywhere that have been proven to cure AIDS, although the search for such drugs is being pursued vigorously. Some drugs have been found that inhibit the AIDS virus, but these have not yet led to clinical improvement. Though no treatment has yet been successful in restoring the immune system of an AIDS patient, doctors have had some success in using drugs, radiation, and surgery to treat the various illnesses of AIDS patients.* Therapeutic agents are needed for all stages of AIDS infections, to block action of the virus once infection has occurred, and to restore full function in patients whose immune systems have been damaged.

Eventually, a combination of therapies to combat the virus and restore the immune system may be the most effective treatment.

Pneumocystis carinii pneumonia, for example, can be treated with antibiotics. Interferon, a virus-fighting protein produced naturally by the body, has been used with some success against Kaposi's sarcoma. Natural and recombinant interleukin preparations are being used in an attempt to repair the immunologic deficiencies in AIDS patients.

Can AIDS be prevented?

Yes. Cases of AIDS related to medical use of blood or blood products are being prevented by use of HTLV-III antibody screening tests at blood donor sites and by members of high risk groups voluntarily not donating blood. Heat treatment of Factor VIII and other blood products helps prevent AIDS in patients with hemophilia and other clotting disorders. There is no vaccine for AIDS itself. However, there is good reason to believe that individuals can reduce their risk of contracting AIDS by following existing recommendations. Communities can help prevent AIDS by vigorous efforts to educate and inform their populations about the illness, with special emphasis on educational activities for members of high risk groups. Meanwhile, the discovery of the AIDS virus and methods developed for producing large

*See editor's note at the end of this reading.

quantities of the virus for experimental and other purposes enables scientists to work at developing a vaccine.

The Public Health Service recommends that the following steps be taken to prevent the spread of AIDS:

- Do not have sexual intercourse with AIDS patients, with members of the risk groups, or with people who are positive for the AIDS virus. If you do, use a condom and avoid sexual practices that may injure tissue.
- Do not use IV drugs. If you do, do not share needles. Don't have sex with people who use IV drugs.
- Women who are sex partners of risk group members or who use IV drugs should consider the risk to their babies *before* pregnancy. These women should have an HTLV-III antibody test before pregnancy. If they elect to become pregnant, they should have a test during pregnancy.
- Do not have sex with multiple partners, including prostitutes (who may also be IV drug abusers). The more partners you have, the greater your chances of catching AIDS.
- People at increased risk for AIDS should not donate blood, organs or sperm.

People with positive HTLV-III antibody tests should observe the following additional recommendations:

- A regular medical evaluation, followup and counseling should be sought.
- Do not donate blood, sperm or organs.
- Do not share drugs with others, and avoid exchanging body fluids during sexual activity (a condom should be used). Avoid oral-genital contact and intimate kissing.
- Do not share toothbrushes, razors or other implements that could become contaminated with blood.
- Observe the recommendations on pregnancy.

Further information about AIDS may be obtained from your local or State health department or your physician. The Public Health Service AIDS hotline number is 1-800-342-AIDS. Atlanta area callers should dial (404)329-1295.

(**Editor's note:** In September 1986, federal health officials announced that an experimental drug has been shown to have prolonged AIDS patients survival. It is a promising new drug called azidothymidine (AZT), but officials stress that it is not a cure, even though it has prolonged life.)

OVERVIEW

THE COST OF AIDS

Peter S. Arno

Despite medical breakthroughs in isolating and describing the probable causative agent in AIDS and some basic advances in immunology and virology, vaccine development and fundamental control of the AIDS epidemic appear to be years away. . . .

It is likely that the AIDS epidemic will place increasingly greater strains upon the health care system in cities and countries with a large number of cases of AIDS, as well as on both public and private sources of health care financing. The problem will intensify as the epidemic continues to grow, particularly in high-incidence areas such as New York, San Francisco, Los Angeles and Miami, which together account for approximately 60 percent of the nation's total reported cases. In addition, while the absolute number of AIDS cases continues to grow in high-incidence metropolitan areas, there is convincing evidence that it is spreading geographically across the country. . . .

Peter S. Arno is an economist at the Institute for Health Policy Studies and the Aging Health Policy Center at the University of California in San Fransisco. His comments were excerpted from a hearing by the House Subcommittee on Health and the Environment, July 22, 1985.

Cost Estimates

Despite the seriousness of the AIDS epidemic and its exponential spread throughout the nation, information and published data on the costs of treatment of AIDS patients is practically non-existent. In the literature, two cost estimates have been reported. The first, published in the *Annals of Internal Medicine* in August 1983 by Groopman and Detsky, estimates the cost of treatment at between $50,000 and $100,000 per patient. However, the basis of this estimate is not stated, nor are the figures broken down in further detail. A more recent estimate was published in the February 21, 1985 issue of the *New England Journal of Medicine* by Landesman, Ginzburg and Weiss. They estimate the average direct lifetime cost of an AIDS patient to be $42,000. However, this figure is based on a study of 16 patients; as we all know, a comprehensive cost analysis requires a far larger sample size.

In a preliminary cost analysis of the first 9000 AIDS cases in the United States, Hardy and her associates at the Centers for Disease Control, U.S. Public Health Service, estimated a cost of $140,000 per patient. The hospital costs were calculated by multiplying the total number of hospital days by the average daily charge for AIDS patients. . .

All of the costs discussed above are for inpatient stays at hospitals only. They do not reflect the cost of outpatient visits to private physicians or clinics or the array of social support and counseling services that are provided largely through the voluntary non-profit sector. (We are in the process of assessing these costs and will report on them in the future.) Furthermore, an often neglected dimension of the economic impact of illness on society is the indirect costs associated with the loss of one's social contribution to society's production of goods and services. This is particularly severe in the case of AIDS because most victims are struck down in the prime of their life. In Hardy's study, the indirect costs of AIDS were measured in terms of work years lost due to disability and premature death. For the first 9,000 cases of AIDS it was estimated that approximately 7,538 years of work due to disability were lost at a cost of 162 million dollars as well as 4.2 billion dollars in future earnings due to premature death. Thus, in total, more than 4.3

$6.3 Billion

The cost of the nation's first 10,000 cases of AIDS will come to more than $6.3 billion in hospital fees and lost income, according to a study thought to be the first to estimate the economic impact of the disease. . . .It is estimated that approximately $147,000 is being expended for the hospital care of each patient with AIDS," researchers said.

Minneapolis Star and Tribune, *1986*

billion dollars have been lost in indirect costs (Hardy et al., 1985). While these figures are quite rough they do indicate the magnitude of the indirect economic loss due to the AIDS epidemic.

Scitovsky Study

The data that I would like to report was gathered and analyzed in a study done under the direction of Anne Scitovsky of the Palo Alto Medical Foundation and the Institute for Health Policy Studies of the University of California, San Francisco, with Mary Cline, Philip Lee and myself. I will present some of the preliminary findings from our detailed study on the cost of inpatient treatment of AIDS patients at San Francisco General Hospital (SFGH), where approximately 30 percent of San Francisco's AIDS patients are treated.

We secured data on charges for 311 out of 330 admissions of AIDS patients to SFGH during the period January through September 1984. The data include charges for hospital services and professional fees for surgical and anesthetist services. The data on professional fees came from the final bills while the data on hospital charges came from the discharge summary bills which are not necessarily the final bills. However, we believe that our data understate actual charges by no more than five percent. . . .

Our estimate of the total cost of lifetime in-hospital treatment for AIDS ranges between $25,000 and $32,000 per patient in San Francisco. . . .

A final point regarding the availability and accessibility of outpatient and community-based care facilities and programs in San Francisco, and the relatively low charges per admission at SFGH as compared to elsewhere, may give us an important clue to the direction we should follow in a rational planning policy for the treatment of AIDS patients. The average length of stay at SFGH, at 11.4 days, is far shorter than in other cities. This may be due in part to the different patient mix, type of opportunistic infections and practice patterns that are found in various parts of the country. However, it should be recognized that the availability and accessibility of outpatient clinics, home health and hospice care, and other social support services, while not ideal in San Francisco, do allow patients to be discharged from the hospital earlier than in other cities where such services are not as readily available. . . .

We believe the investment of public funds in these community-based services not only affords better quality care, but also is cost-effective and reduces the need for inpatient hospital care—saving private health insurance expenditures, Medicaid expenditures and local tax revenues that must be spent for inpatient care when Medicaid or other third-party reimbursement is below costs. . . .

Conclusion

Let me conclude with a brief comment on the implications of the cost data that I have presented. It is very clear that the AIDS epidemic continues unabated. . . .

In San Francisco we estimate the total lifetime costs of inpatient hospital treatment to be between $25,000 and $32,000 per patient. The CDC has estimated the costs to be $143,000 per patient, or $1.25 billion annually just for hospital inpatient care. Currently perhaps as many as one-third or more of AIDS patients are covered by Medicaid—an indication that they have lost their health insurance due to their loss of employment related to illness or that they were uninsured.

The problem of paying for health care is particularly tragic for AIDS patients because they must confront catastrophic health care costs when they are least able to pay. In the current climate of competition, deregulation and decentralization—or abrogation of federal responsibility, as I believe it

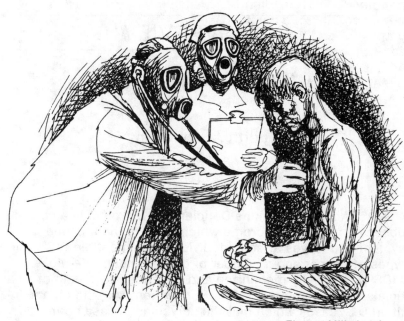

Eleanor Mill sketch

should more appropriately be designated—the AIDS victim must spend down his resources, pauperize himself and then apply for public assistance. Only in the United States of America and South Africa, among all western industrialized nations, would such a fate befall a sick patient with catastrophic health care costs.

The key question—for AIDS patients, as well as for all Americans—is what is the federal government's role in health care financing? The failure of the federal government to meet its responsibilities doesn't eliminate the costs of health care; it simply shifts them to other levels of government (increasingly local government) and to individuals. In the past the costs could also be shifted to private health insurance, through cost shifting within hospitals. That day is rapidly passing and we will soon have to face the question of how best to finance health care for all Americans.

OVERVIEW

AIDS IN AMERICA

Judith A. Johnson

AIDS (Acquired Immune Deficiency Syndrome) is a newly observed medical syndrome which impairs the immune system and leaves affected individuals susceptible to certain types of cancer and a number of opportunistic infections. AIDS was initially recognized and described by health officials in the summer of 1981. Subsequent investigation identified U.S. cases which met the surveillance case definition and which were under medical care as early as 1975. The mortality rate of AIDS is extremely high; 75% of AIDS patients diagnosed prior to January 1984 are now deceased. The Centers for Disease Control (CDC), the National Institutes of Health (NIH), the Food and Drug Administration (FDA), and the Alcohol Drug Abuse and Mental Health Administration (ADAMHA) are funding research on the cause and treatment of AIDS.

As of March 3, 1986, 17,871 definite cases of AIDS have been reported to the Centers for Disease Control (CDC) from all 50 States, Puerto Rico, and the District of Columbia. Fifty-six percent of AIDS cases were reported to be residents of New York City, NY; San Francisco, CA; Miami, FL; Newark, NJ; or Los Angeles, CA. Forty-five States, the District of Columbia, and Puerto Rico now require physicians to report cases of AIDS to State or local health departments.

Judith A. Johnson is a science policy research specialist for the Library of Congress. Her comments were excerpted from a Library of Congress publication titled *AIDS: Acquired Immune Deficiency Syndrome,* March 7, 1986.

AIDS in San Francisco

San Francisco has the second largest number of AIDS cases, and the highest per capita rate in the Nation. Up to this date, we have had approximately 700 cases and 300 deaths; last month alone, there were 50 cases diagnosed and 28 deaths.

Congressional Testimony by Mervyn Silverman, M.D., September, 1984

As of March 3, 1986, 254 cases of AIDS in children have been reported to the CDC; of the 254, 152 are now dead. All had opportunistic infections or Kaposi's sarcoma. The majority of the children have parents who either are AIDS patients or are at risk of contracting AIDS (i.e., intravenous drug abuser), or the child had received a blood transfusion. CDC had originally been reluctant to include children on the list of known AIDS cases because they may possibly have had an inherited immune disorder. However, none of the childhood cases fits the symptoms of any well-characterized inherited immune defect. Children are now included in the figures CDC provides for totals of AIDS cases. There has been some speculation that the children may have acquired the disease from routine household contact with an infected adult, but it is more probable that it was acquired *in utero* or through intimate contact, as occurs between mother and child. On August 30, 1985, CDC issued recommendations on education and foster care of children infected with the HTLV-III virus.

HTLV-III and the HTLV-III Antibody Test

On March 2, 1985, HHS Secretary Margaret M. Heckler announced the FDA approval of an HTLV-III blood test developed by Abbott Laboratories; shortly afterward, the FDA also approved tests developed by Electro-Nucleonics and Litton Bionetics. Under the licensing agreement, the Federal Government will receive 5% of the net revenue from sales of the test, which could run as high as $150 million annually. . . .

On January 10, 1985, the U.S. Public Health Service issued provisional recommendations for administering the AIDS test. The recommendations are contained in the Jan. 11, 1985, issue of the Morbidity and Mortality Weekly Report. All donated blood will be tested and donors will be notified if their tests are positive. The names of donors with positive tests will be placed on the collection facility's donor deferral list and may be added to additional deferral lists as required by 21 CFR 606.160(e). This procedure also occurs with other infectious diseases, such as hepatitis B. Blood that tests positive will not be used in transfusions or manufactured into other products. The test will be repeated before the donor is notified.

Since many high-risk individuals may want to be tested, the test will also be available through private physicians, health centers, and public health clinics. CDC (Center for Disease Control) has provided $9.7 million to help State and local governments set up such "alternative testing sites". (New England Journal of Medicine, Oct. 31, 1985, p. 1158.) However, because the test will only detect antibody to HTLV-III in the blood, it will not provide clear information about whether the persons being tested will develop AIDS or whether they have merely been exposed to the virus and have mounted a successful immune response.

Of the 1.1 million units of blood collected at 155 centers from implementation of the test in the spring of 1985 through June 16, 1985, 2,831, or 0.25%, had a positive HTLV-III antibody test. Of these, approximately one-third, 0.08% of the total, or one per 1,200 donors, were also positive on a second type of test, the "Western blot," suggesting that they were infected with HTLV-III. . . .

AIDS Transmission via Blood Products

Reports of hemophilia-associated AIDS in the U.S. were first published in July 1982. As of Feb. 10, 1986, 149 hemophiliacs have acquired AIDS. Hemophiliacs require two to three injections per week of a blood clotting factor, factor VIII, as part of the treatment for their genetic disease. A hemophiliac using factor VIII may be exposed to the blood of 25,000 to 75,000 people every year, and a given donor may potentially expose approximately 100 recipients of the con-

AIDS in New York City

We have had 2,995 cases of AIDS in New York City to date. We don't know how many people are infected in New York, but the best estimates say there are at least a half a million people in New York City who are gay. Serologic surveys in certain circumstances have shown that half of the gay population may be infected with AIDS. That means in New York City 250,000 gay people are potentially infected.

There are 190,000 current IV drug abusers in New York City. One study that was done in New York City showed 80 percent of the IV drug abusers are infected with the HTLV-III virus. So, I think the estimate of 300,000 to 400,000 in the country is perhaps an understatement. We have that many probably in New York City alone.

To date, 1,573 people have died of AIDS. The average age of death of these people is 39 years of age. In New York City if you live to be 35, you should go on and live to be 79. AIDS is a young people's disease.

David J. Sencer, M.D., New York City Health Commissioner, February, 1985

centrated blood-clotting factor. In March 1983, FDA announced its approval of a heat treatment which kills hepatitis B virus in factor VIII preparations. It is hoped that the treatment will also inactivate the AIDS virus.

As of Feb. 10, 1986, CDC had received reports of 316 cases of AIDS in individuals who received blood transfusions. Research studies on transfusion-associated AIDS indicate that exposure to as little as one unit of blood may result in the transmission of AIDS. Most donors in transfusion-associated AIDS cases apparently had only mild or inapparent illness at the time of blood donation. Three million Americans, including 15,000 hemophiliacs, receive blood or blood products each year. It is expected that the

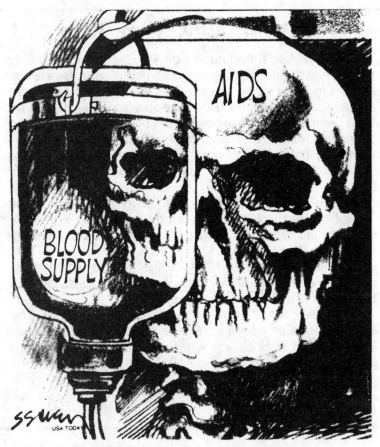

implementation of the AIDS antibody test in the spring of 1985 will prevent the further transmission of AIDS through blood transfusion. However, since the incubation period between exposure to the virus and development of the disease may be as long as 5 years, CDC expects that such cases will continue to be reported for the next several years.

Treatment of AIDS

At the present time there is no known cure for AIDS. Three different approaches are being used in the treatment of AIDS patients: (1) treat the opportunistic infection or cancer that is currently affecting the patient; (2) treat the AIDS virus itself;

and (3) stimulate the patient's immune system. The first approach is only palliative, since it does not eliminate the underlying cause of the patient's disease. Certain drugs have had limited success in reducing or eliminating Kaposi's sarcoma lesions and in treating the other forms of cancer and some of the opportunistic infections that affect these patients. However, since the treatment does not enable AIDS patients to regain the function of their immune system, the opportunistic infections or cancer will eventually recur. The opportunistic infections are particularly difficult to treat and for some illnesses there is no known treatment.

Examples of drugs used to treat the opportunistic infections and cancers that afflict AIDS patients are the following: DFMO, Fansidar, DHPG, spiramycin, clofazimine, rifampin, Pentamidine, trimethoprimsulfamethoxazole and vincristine.

The second approach attempts to make use of anti-viral drugs in order to inhibit the AIDS virus. Although new anti-viral drugs are continuing to be developed, unfortunately only a small number of useful anti-viral agents are available at the present time. . . .

Examples of anti-viral drugs being tested for use in the treatment of AIDS (and in certain cases AIDS-related complex) are the following: foscarnet (PFA, phosphonoformate), HPA-23, Virazole (ribavirin), AZT (azidothymidine, Compound S, BW A509U), suramin, ansamycin, and AL721. In general, the anti-viral drugs tested to date do not significantly improve the clinical status of the AIDS patient even though they appear to suppress the activities of the virus. The drugs are quite toxic, and the virus reappears when treatment is stopped.

Even if the appropriate anti-viral drug is discovered, the drug must be administered before the patient's immune system is beyond repair. Additional therapy in the form of immune system stimulants or bone marrow transplantation may be required in order to restore the immune system. This is the third approach to AIDS treatment mentioned earlier in this section.

Examples of drugs affecting the immune system that are being tested on AIDS are the following: alpha interferon, gamma interferon, IMREG-1, interleukin-2, isoprinosine, imuthiol, and cyclosporine. Several have been tried in AIDS

The Future of AIDS

Tenfold Increase

To date, the government has recorded 21,517 cases of AIDS and 11,713 deaths from the disease, which destroys the body's resistance. The Public Health Service estimated that by the end of 1991 there would be a cumulative total of 270,000 cases and 179,000 deaths.

New York Times, *June, 1986*

Drug Use Spreading AIDS

A federal official responsible for battling AIDS has warned that cases linked to intravenous drug use, once concentrated in two states are rapidly spreading throughout the nation.

He said that swift action must be taken to stem a further spread of the disease by this means and that intravenous drug use is now viewed as a far greater factor in the spread of AIDS than had been realized.

Minneapolis Star and Tribune, *April 6, 1986*

AIDS in Infants

AIDS has become the most common infectious disease in newborn infants in some parts of New York City, spreading increasingly rapidly among children even as the adult AIDS epidemic slows. . . .

As of Jan. 13, 1986, 231 cases of AIDS in infants had been reported to the federal Centers for Disease Control in Atlanta. About 40 percent of them, or 103 cases occurred in New York City. . . .

Most of the children are born to mothers who are intravenous drug abusers and thus are at high risk of contracting AIDS from the sharing of needles.

Associated Press, 1986

patients with little or no clinical success. Researchers are hoping that perhaps these drugs in combination with the anti-virals will have a better chance of success than either has alone against the AIDS virus to date. Clinical trials using a combination therapy, however, will need more time and patients than trials of a single drug therapy in order to determine optimal timing of drug delivery as well as safe and effective drug dosage levels.

Treating the patient early in the course of the disease, before the immune system has been destroyed, may offer the best hope for recovery. However, since the incubation period of the disease may be as long as 5 or 6 years and is often asymptomatic, it may be difficult to determine when treatment should begin and for how long it should be continued. In addition, not all of the individuals exposed to the virus would be candidates for early therapy since only one-third of this group is now thought to go on to develop AIDS. Because prolonged treatment and observation of the patient will probably be necessary in order to control the AIDS virus and reconstitute the immune system, and because such treatments will involve toxic side effects, it will be necessary to use great care in patient selection for clinical trials.

OVERVIEW

AIDS IN PRISONS AND JAILS

Theodore M. Hammett

In the correctional context, dealing with the problem of AIDS may pose even more difficult problems since inmate populations may include high proportions of individuals in AIDS risk groups, particularly intravenous drug users. Correctional administrators must formulate policies that allow them to manage their institutions effectively, while dealing with a serious health problem that may cause fears among staff and inmates. Administrators face difficult decisions concerning prevention, housing, and the provision of medical care, decisions which are frequently complicated by legal and cost issues. . . .

In response to urgent information needs expressed by corrections professionals, the National Institute of Justice and the American Correctional Association sponsored a study entitled *AIDS in Correctional Facilties: Issues and Options.* The study was based, in large part, on responses to a national mail questionnaire from all 50 State correctional departments, the Federal Bureau of Prisons, and 33 large city and county jail systems. The responses were received between November 1985 and January 1986.

AIDS in the Correctional Population

Responses to the study questionnaire reveal that, since 1981, there have been a cumulative total of 455 confirmed AIDS cases in 25 State and Federal prison systems. Twenty large city and county jail systems reported 311 cases of

Theodore M. Hammett, "Aids in Prisons and Jails," *Issues in Brief,* National Institute of Justice, February, 1986, pp. 1-8.

AIDS among inmates. These figures represent *cumulative* total cases since the responding jurisdictions began keeping records.

As of the period November 1985 to January 1986, there were 144 cases of AIDS among State and Federal inmates in 19 systems and 35 cases among city and county inmates in 11 systems.

No known AIDS cases have occurred among correctional staff as a result of contact with inmates. Questionaire respondents reported nine cases of AIDS among current or former staff, but none of these individuals had been involved in an incident with an inmate in which transmission of the AIDS virus might have occurred. Indeed, most were known or suspected to have been in AIDS risk groups.

The distribution of AIDS cases across correctional systems is highly skewed. Fifty-one percent of the prision systems have had *no* cases and 80 percent have had fewer than four cases. Among responding city and county jail systems, 39 percent have had no cases and 70 percent have had fewer than four cases.

At the other extreme, two State prison systems and only one of the responding city and county jail systems have had more than 50 cases. The regional distribution is also highly uneven. Over 70 percent of the cases, both in State prison systems and in city and county jail systems, have occurred in the mid-Atlantic region, with all other parts of the United States contributing much smaller percentages.

The vast majority of correctional AIDS cases, particularly in jurisdictions with large numbers of cases, are believed to be associated with prior intravenous drug abuse. There is substantial debate, but little hard data, on the extent to which the AIDS virus is being transmitted within correctional institutions. The two primary means of transmission are pro-hibited behavior in all corrections systems. However, logic and common sense suggest that, even in the best-managed correctional facilities, there may be at least some transmission of the infection occurring among inmates. . . .

HTLV-III Antibody Testing

There is substantial debate, both in corrections and in society at large, surrounding the uses of the HTLV-III antibody test and the meaning of the test results. The most controversial testing application in corrections is mass screening: the testing of all inmates or all new inmates, regardless of the presence of symptoms or other clinical indications.

Correctional Policies on HTLV-III Antibody Testing

Only four State correctional systems (Nevada, Colorado, Iowa, and Missouri) have implemented or plan to implement mass screening programs for inmates; no city or county systems responding to the questionnaire have instituted or planned such programs. However, almost 90 percent of the responding jurisdictions do employ testing for more limited purposes. These include testing of risk-group members, testing in support of diagnoses of AIDS or ARC, testing in response to incidents in which the AIDS virus might have been transmitted, testing on inmate request, and testing carried out as part of anonymous epidemiological studies.

Correctional Management Issues

Ironically, the medical treatment of AIDS patients may be the simplest issue confronting correctional administrators. Other questions—where to house and treat the inmate, how to prevent the spread of the disease, and how to pay for medical care—are likely to be even more difficult to resolve.

Housing policies. One of the most critical and difficult decisions for correctional administrators is where to house and treat inmates wilth AIDS, ARC, or HTLV-III seropositivity. Of course, medical considerations dictate many of these decisions. Most jurisdictions place inmates with confirmed diagnoses of AIDS in a medical facility either within the correctional system or in the community, although the duration of such hospitalization varies considerably.

Preventing the spread of AIDS within the prison and protecting affected inmates from intimidation and violence are important considerations. Other factors in treatment and housing decisions include availability and location of facilities able to provide appropriate care, costs of any new construction or renovations necessary to prepare special units, and staffing of any special AIDS units (correctional as well as medical).

Correctional administrators have a number of options concerning treatment and housing placements for inmates with AIDS, ARC, or HTLV-III seropositivity. The key options are the following:

1. maintaining inmates in the general population;
2. returning inmates to the general population when their illnesses are in remission;
3. administratively segregating inmates in a separate unit or relying on single-cell housing;
4. hospitalization; and
5. case-by-case determination of all housing and treatment decisions. . . .

Notification and confidentiality. One of the most difficult and sensitive issues regarding AIDS in corrections is who receives information on the medical status of inmates with AIDS, ARC, or HTLV-III seropositivity. Decisions regarding who should receive HTLV-III antibody test results and who should be notified of AIDS or ARC diagnoses may be dictated by precise legal and policy standards such as requirements for written authorization to release test results or other medical records. . . .

Where law or policy allows any discretion, decisions regarding disclosure versus confidentiality invariably raise the question of which should take precedence; the inmate's right to have medical information kept confidential or the correctional system's perceived legal and moral responsibility to protect its staff and other inmates, as well as the public, from HTLV-III infection. . . .

The most compelling reason for maintaining confidentiality is that persons known to have AIDS, ARC, or HTLV-III seropositivity may suffer ostracism, threats, and possibly violent intimidation while in prison, and discrimination in employment, housing, and insurance availability after they are discharged.

Because of their rapid population turnover rates, jails face even more difficult policy decisions and logistical problems regarding disclosure and confidentiality of medical information. . . .

Costs of care and associated services. Questionnaire responses showed that correctional systems are almost universally concerned about the costs of medical care and associated services for inmates with AIDS. Questions regarding range of costs elicited widely varying estimates, but all agreed that medical care for AIDS patients is extremely expensive, whether it is provided in a correctional medical facility, in another public medical facility, or in a hospital in the community, particularly because correctional inmates are ineligible for Medicaid reimbursement.

Correctional systems should plan on spending anywhere from $40,000 to over $600,000 for hospitalization and associated medical costs of caring for each inmate with AIDS. The costs will vary depending on the amount of acute care required; they will also probably be higher if inmates are placed in hospitals in the community than if they are retained in correctional medical facilities or other public medical facilities.

To the figures for hospitalization and medical care must be added costs of ancillary services such as counseling, possible legal assistance, increased insurance (unless the system is self-insured), and funerals. Obviously, medical care and associated services for inmates with AIDS could have serious budgetary implications for correctional systems.

AIDS poses complex and difficult problems for correctional systems. The only certainty is that the problems will not disappear. Every correctional system should develop comprehensive policies and procedures for managing the AIDS problem in its institutions. The information provided here and in the full report can help correctional administrators consider the range of options available and the strengths and weaknesses of each.

OVERVIEW

AIDS SPREADING AMONG HETEROSEXUALS IN AFRICA

Lawrence K. Altman

AIDS appears to be spreading by conventional sexual intercourse among heterosexuals in Africa and is striking women nearly as often as men, according to researchers here.

These scientists are involved in two related battles: controlling the incurable disease and fighting suppression of information crucial to the international search for its origin, cause and cure.

Perhaps of greatest long-term importance in Africa, where birthrates are booming, is that a continued unchecked spread of AIDS among sexually active women has caused many babies to be born with the disease and could lead to many more such births. The AIDS virus can pass from mother to fetus in pregnancy and through breast milk to an infant after birth.

Major Mystery

Why the pattern of communicability seems to differ so drastically in Africa from that elsewhere is one of the major mysteries of one of the most confounding medical stories of this century.

Medical scientists believe that far more research, testing and reporting on the disease in Africa need to be done before those patterns can be fully understood and before any conclusions can be drawn from them.

Africa has been the focus of attention for some time, in part because some scientists have suggested that the disease may have originated there. However, others point out that it was first recognized, not in Africa, but in the United States, and that no scientific evidence has proved any theories about where it originated.

But what is clear is that the disorder has become a major public health concern in Central Africa, that it is emerging as one in East Africa and that scientists now generally believe the African experience, however it is ultimately diagnosed, will almost certainly contain lessons vital to the health of people throughout the world.

AIDS Transmission

The epidemiology of AIDS in Africa, where homosexuality does not seem to be common, contrasts radically with findings elsewhere. Except for Haiti, AIDS has occurred in other areas of the world mostly among homosexual men, although some experts are concerned that it may become an increasing risk among heterosexuals there as well.

In the United States, more than 70% of the more than 14,500 AIDS victims have been homosexual or bisexual men. Federal authorities attribute only 1% of the nation's AIDS cases to intimate heterosexual contact, and nearly all these cases involve women who were apparently infected with the AIDS virus through sexual contact with an infected man.

Acquired immune deficiency syndrome, or AIDS, which was discovered in 1981, has been known to be a worldwide public health problem since 1983, and there has been increasing recognition of the dimensions of the problem in recent months. The number of countries reporting AIDS to the World Health Organization in Geneva jumped to 71 in October from 40 in August, with the case count nearing 17,000.

Although individual doctors have reported in various medical journals on AIDS cases among residents of almost 20 countries in Africa, no country in Central, East or West Africa has reported any cases to the World Health Organization. So it is not possible to obtain an accurate total count of cases on the continent. South Africa does report to the international agency.

To this reporter, who is also a physician and who has examined AIDS patients and interviewed dozens of doctors

AIDS in Africa Spreads Among Heterosexuals

According to the most reliable reports, AIDS in Africa seems to be primarily a heterosexual disease because it affects men and women in equal numbers, while the U.S. ratio is about 15 men to every woman. Says Haseltine in arguing that AIDS is fast becoming a heterosexual disease, "To think that we're so different from people in the Congo is a nice, comfortable position, but it probably isn't so. It's heterosexual promiscuity. The more lovers, the better the chance of being infected.". . .

Johns Hopkins professor of medicine Frank Polk cautions against assuming that AIDS in Africa is spread only through heterosexual contact. He recently returned from a research trip to central Africa, and he believes that homosexuality is more common there than officials care to admit. . . .

Polk is also quick to emphasize the role that contaminated needles may have played in the spread of AIDS in Africa. "I suspect that up to half of all AIDS cases there are probably the result of needles that have been re-used in health clinics, and needles used in certain tribal customs," he says. Infectious disease expert Thomas Quinn of Johns Hopkins adds that in poor countries the cost of disposable needles and syringes limits their availability.

Discover, *December, 1985*

while traveling through Africa, the disease is clearly a more important public health problem than many African governments acknowledge. In trying to explain the dimensions of the problem, and his frustrations in dealing with it, one physician picked up two thick packs of green hospital record charts, one for AIDS cases, the other for suspected cases, and said quietly: "They are growing thicker each week."

Yet, he said, the director of the hospital has told him to tell officials that he has diagnosed only two cases of the disease.

Accurate Information

Access to accurate information has been shut off in many cases. Some expatriates working in Central and East Africa have said they feel threatened with expulsion from their host countries if they talk freely without government approval. Some African countries have refused visas to journalists inquiring about AIDS.

And in at least one government, according to Western diplomatic sources, a rift has developed between ministries that want to suppress information about AIDS and health officials who, in the absence of effective treatments and vaccines, are eager to provide more public education to stall the epidemic.

In some important ways, Rwanda is a notable exception to the suppression of information. Its doctors have been permitted to publish in journals and grant a limited number of interviews. According to new data provided by one expert, the number of cases in Rwanda, although an incomplete total, has surged each year since 1982 in a pattern similar to that in the U.S. and elsewhere. Most cases have occurred in Kigali, the capital, with a preponderance among those in the middle and upper class. About 40% of the cases have been among women.

The total number of AIDS cases has risen sharply since 1982, when a single case was reported. There were six reported cases in 1983, 86 in 1984 and 224 so far this year.

Children accounted for 70 of these 317 cases, or 22%, a proportion that contrasts sharply with that of the United States. The Centers for Disease Control in Atlanta reports that children accounted for only 206 of the 14,519 AIDS cases in the United States, or 1.4% of the total.

The childhood afflictions in Rwanda and elsewhere in Africa are of particular concern to medical researchers. "Since nearly half the cases of AIDS in Africa occur among women in their reproductive years, and since these women are having many babies, perinatal transmission is a very important problem," said Peter Piot, a professor of microbiology at the Institute of Tropical Medicine in Antwerp, Belgium, who is helping coordinate African research projects on AIDS.

Thus, there is the potential of a possible health menace of staggering proportions for future generations of Africans.

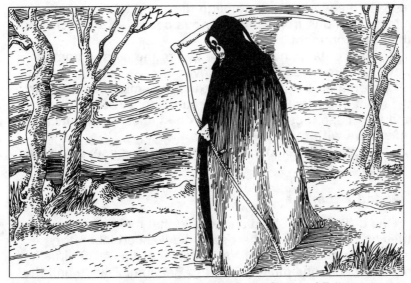

Reprinted by permission of the *Minneapolis Star and Tribune*

Nevertheless, the secretary general of the Rwandan Ministry of Health, Francois-Xavier Hakizimana, says the disease, although a threat, is not at present the No. 1 public health concern. "We prefer to talk about malaria, diarrhea and parasitic diseases and malnutrition, which are our major public health problems," he said in an interview.

He said his government had added AIDS to its educational programs against sexually transmitted diseases, although it did not plan a specific campaign against AIDS.

The importance of public education is underscored by the supposition among physicians in Africa that just one conventional sexual encounter may be sufficient to transmit AIDS, if one is to believe the sexual histories that patients have given their doctors. However, the risk of AIDS appears to increase with the number of different sexual partners.

The Same Disease

Scientists believe that although the communicable nature of AIDS in Africa is markedly different from what it is in the rest of the world, the disease itself is the same. They come to that conclusion primarily because the virus HTLVIII-LAV seems to be equally incriminated as the cause of the disease the world over, although they can detect seemingly minor variations from within various countries and from continent to continent.

Sexual contact and blood are two of the most common ways AIDS is spread the world over.

Doctors here regard heterosexual transmission as by far the most important factor in the spread of AIDS in Africa, and they base these conclusions on studies of victims and interviews with them and their families.

The possibility exists that unadmitted homosexuality may be a factor.

Needed Expertise

One difficulty in blood analysis is that most of these countries do not have the expertise and advanced laboratory equipment needed to test for evidence of the AIDS virus in blood. Specimens must be sent to Belgium, France and the United States for virus testing, which, although a slow process, eventually does help in overall research findings.

But the consequence of the lack of proper testing is that AIDS-contaminated blood may often be transfused every day into patients who for various reasons are in need of donated blood. According to one study of about 100 donors in Rwanda, 20% had antibodies to the virus and presumably could pass on the virus.

OVERVIEW

SEXUAL AILMENTS POSING COLOSSAL WORLDWIDE THREAT

Associated Press

Sexually transmitted diseases have been around since the beginning of recorded history but now they are posing a health threat on a colossal scale around the globe.

The diseases are so prevalent that people have come to refer to them only by the initials STD. Their consequences range from pain and embarrassment to infant brain damage, cancer and death. Millions of people around the world are infected.

The most frightening STD also is the newest: AIDS, which has killed about 6,000 people in the United States and spread throughout the world since it first was identified in 1981.

But AIDS is only one of about 25 contagious diseases classified as STD. Others include herpes, chlamydia, genital warts, hepatitis B, gonorrhea and syphilis. All can lead to serious complications, especially in babies born to infected women.

While surveillance campaigns in the 1970s have reduced the prevalence of gonorrhea and syphilis in the West, the newer STD are spreading at an alarming rate, specialists said.

"The new world of STD is chlamydia and AIDS and herpes and human papilloma virus (genital warts) and the long term consequences of pelvic infection, ectopic pregnancy, infertility and cervical cancer," said Dr. Ward Cates, director of the STD Division of the Centers for Disease Control in Atlanta.

This month, about 600 doctors and researchers from 40 countries attended a meeting of the International Society for STD Research in England. With about 12,000 reported cases of AIDS in the United States and 940 cases in Europe and with those numbers doubling every nine months, discussion of the disease dominated the meeting's first day. Fourteen papers were presented on the prevalence and treatment of AIDS, or acquired immune deficiency syndrome, which destroys the body's natural immunity to infection. But no one suggested breakthroughs in the search for a cure, prevention or treatment of AIDS.

Evidence from central Africa, where AIDS may have originated, shows that it can be transmitted heterosexually. In the United States and Western Europe, 73 percent of the victims have been homosexual or bisexual males, but in central Africa as many women as men have contracted the disease.

Professor Peter Piot of the Institute of Tropical Medicine in Antwerp, Belgium, said his findings indicate that heterosexual contact is the main way AIDS is being spread in Africa. But he said the phenomenon might be linked to the use of infected needles at hospitals.

Other Diseases

While AIDS poses the greatest danger to the public because there is no cure for it, the disease pales in comparison with other sexually transmitted diseases in terms of the number of people infected.

Cates said 25 million to 40 million Americans have genital warts, a condition linked to cervical cancer, and 15 million to 20 million are infected with one of the four types of herpes, which cause mouth and genital sores and are the commonest cause of congenital mental illness and blindness resulting from a viral infection.

Chlamydia, the No. 1 bacterial sexually transmitted disease, is two to three times more common than gonorrhea. An estimated 3 million to 4 million Americans are believed to be carriers of the disease, which produces no overt symptoms in women. If untreated, chlamydia can cause blindness, infertility and severe eye and chest infections in the newborn.

About 1 million Americans and 200 million people worldwide are believed to carry the viral infection hepatitis B, which can lead to cirrhosis and liver cancer and is a leading cause of death among men in parts of Africa and Asia. The disease is mainly spread nonsexually by infected blood, but it is considered an STD because of a high incidence among male homosexuals.

Dr. George Antal, program manager of STD for the World Health Organization in Geneva, Switzerland, said there were

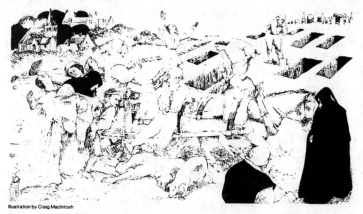

Illustration by Craig MacIntosh

Reprinted by permission of the *Minneapolis Star and Tribune*.

Sexually transmitted diseases

About 12,000 AIDS cases have been reported in the United States since 1981. Here are estimates of the number of sufferers of other sexually transmitted diseases in the U.S. in 1984:

Genital warts	Herpes	Chlamydia	Hepatitis B	Gonorrhea	Syphilis
25-40 million	15-20 million	3-4 million	1 million	879,587	69,886

Source: Dr. Ward Gates, Center for Disease Control, Atlanta

no reliable figures on the worldwide incidence of STD. Some of the STD are not yet listed as reportable communicable diseases in the West, and gonorrhea and syphilis are under-reported in the Third World, he said.

Antal said the best indicator of the spread of STD was a British survey showing an overall rise of 37 percent in the number of new cases seen by National Health Service clinics over the past decade, from 347,000 in 1973 to 547,000 in 1983.

Cates said the rise in sexually transmitted diseases is attributable mainly to the aging of the U.S. baby-boom generation, the tendency for people to stay single longer and increased sexual activity among teen-agers. In addition, there have been advances in detecting the diseases and the use of birth-control pills instead of barrier contraceptives has facilitated the spread of the contagious microorganisms that cause STD.

There are 3,500 STD clinics in the United States, but about half of the patients are treated by private doctors and most of those cases are not reported to the Centers for Disease Control, Cates said.

The drain on health care services is enormous: one study estimated the annual cost of just one aspect of STD — pelvic inflammatory disease caused by chlamydia and gonorrhea — at $2.8 billion a year in health expenses and lost work, he said.

According to the Atlanta centers, cases of gonorrhea in the United States fell 2.9 percent between 1974 and 1984, from 906,121 to 879,587, and the reported incidence of syphilis fell 16.6 percent, from 83,771 to 69,886. As with other such diseases, except for AIDS, Cates said the actual number of cases probably is two times higher than the reported number.

44

RECOGNIZING AUTHOR'S POINT OF VIEW

This activity may be used as an individualized study guide for students in libraries and resource centers or as a discussion catalyst in small group and classroom discussions.

The capacity to recognize an author's point of view is an essential reading skill. Many readers do not make clear distinctions between descriptive articles that relate factual information and articles that express a point of view. Think about the readings in chapter one. Are these readings essentially descriptive articles that relate factual information or articles that attempt to persuade through editorial commentary and analysis?

Guidelines

1. Read through the following source descriptions. Choose one of the source descriptions that best describes each reading in chapter one.

Source Descriptions
   a. **Essentially an article that relates factual information**
   b. **Essentially an article that expresses editorial points of view**
   c. **Both of the above**
   d. **None of the above**

2. After careful consideration, pick out one source that you agree with the most. Be prepared to explain the reasons for your choice in a general class discussion.

CHAPTER 2

THE NATIONAL RESPONSE
TO THE AIDS CRISIS

THE NATIONAL RESPONSE

AN INADEQUATE
FEDERAL RESPONSE

Ted Weiss

Ted Weiss is a democratic Congressman from New York and the chairman of the Intergovernmental Relations and Human Resources Subcommittee.

Points to Consider

1. Why have efforts by the Reagan Administration to combat AIDS been inadequate?
2. How are efforts by the Public Health Service (PHS) described?
3. What comments did the Office of Technology Assessment (OTA) make about the Reagan Administration?

Excerpted from testimony by Ted Weiss before a joint hearing of the Subcommittee on Governmental Operations and the Subcommittee on Energy and Commerce, February 21, 1985.

The administration has consistently refused to provide PHS scientists with the level of resources they indicated was urgently needed to address the AIDS epidemic.

I wish we could begin this hearing with a statement to the American people which would be reassuring and optimistic, but it is difficult to speak of the AIDS epidemic without sounding and feeling alarmed. . . .

No cure or vaccine is available and the Government scientists project that there will be 40,000 new cases in the next 2 years.

AIDS recognizes no geographic boundaries. Cases have been reported in 47 States and in countries throughout the world. The seemingly relentless tragedy continues to deepen with each new life that is lost and with the suffering of each individual that it touches. The health care and social service needs of persons afflicted with AIDS, and their families, continue to grow faster than available financial and human resources.

We all wish that we could legislate a cure for this dreaded disease. But as Members of Congress, we are relegated to only providing the resources for the Public Health Service's research, surveillance, and public education activities.

During the last 4 years the PHS researchers' tireless efforts to unlock the mysteries of this virulent medical crisis have been and continue to be truly extraordinary. In a relatively short period of time, PHS funded scientists have made significant advances, and their work now lays the foundation for solving the many remaining unanswered questions about the disorder.

OTA has found, however, that the administration has consistently refused to provide PHS scientists with the level of resources they indicated was urgently needed to address the AIDS epidemic. Although the Department continues to identify AIDS as its No. 1 health priority, its AIDS budget requests would suggest otherwise.

"It's Really Outrageous"

Rep. Henry Waxman, chairman of the House Energy and Commerce subcommittee on Health and the Environment, said that the congressional appropriation for AIDS research for this fiscal year was $244 million. The administration proposes to reduce these funds by 22 percent to $193 million. In the 1987 fiscal year, the administration proposes $213 million for such research, he said. "They talk about it as an increase, but the increase won't reach the level of the $244 million," Waxman said. "It's a shell game."

The administration's request to Congress for AIDS research in fiscal year 1986 began at $85 million and eventually was raised to $196 million. Congress raised the figure to $244 million.

"It's really outrageous," Waxman said. "I can't understand how the president can propose this kind of budget when he talks as if he believes that AIDS is a national emergency. And without the basic research and educational work, things we should have been doing for years now, the epidemic will continue to grow.

New York Times, *February, 1986*

Instead of requesting additional funds from Congress, the administration's policy has been to sacrifice the budget and staff of other important health programs in order to address the AIDS public health emergency. I believe that the American public is ill-served by trading off one health need for another.

Despite the administration's reticence, AIDS funding has been substantially increased each year, largely because of the strong leadership that the Congress, particularly the Appropriations Committees, has exerted in this area.

But in order to do the job, we have been forced to rely on unofficial sources and leaks, an unreliable means of collecting budget information. Clearly this is an unacceptable way for the Federal Government to carry out its responsibilities on any issue, but particularly when faced with possibly the most serious epidemic of modern times.

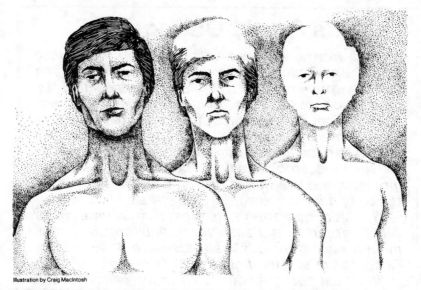

Illustration by Craig MacIntosh

Reprinted by permission of the *Minneapolis Star and Tribune*.

OTA raises other serious concerns for the Congress and the administration to consider. They conclude that confidentiality safeguards for those involved in AIDS research or tested for exposure to HTLV-III can be improved without sacrificing the legitimate data needs of public health officials.

In addition, OTA has found that providing clinical and social services for AIDS patients is already a significant problem that is certain to worsen as the number of AIDS cases increases.

As I read the OTA report in the last few days, I was left with the sad reality that we may be a long, long way from solving the AIDS epidemic. We have no cure, no vaccine, and more questions than answers about a disease that will strike tens of thousands more people.

While I wish that the truly remarkable discovery of HTLV-III was the sought after solution, it actually "only begins the next phase of efforts to control the epidemic." There remains much to do, perhaps years of research, before we halt the spread of AIDS and find a cure for those already suffering. I know all of us here share that goal.

The AIDS Budget

Even conservative estimates suggest that by the early 1990s AIDS will have killed more Americans than died in the Vietnam War. Those frightening predictions point to the need for a massive federal effort to prevent the spread of AIDS, treat its symptoms and find a cure.

The Reagan administration has been reprehensibly slow to comprehend that need. After AIDS was first recognized in 1981, the administration turned down repeated requests by the Centers for Disease Control for additional research money. A turnaround came only last year, when the administration finally bowed to public pressure and boosted AIDS funding to $244 million for fiscal year 1986.

The new budget snatches away that victory by asking Congress to rescind $41 million of the 1986 AIDS appropriation. And the administration's 1987 budget proposes only $213 million—far less than experts predict will be needed.

Minneapolis Star and Tribune, *February 10, 1986*

THE NATIONAL RESPONSE

PROGRESS IN THE BATTLE AGAINST AIDS

James O. Mason

James O. Mason made the following statement in his capacity as Assistant Secretary of Health for the Department of Health and Human Services.

Points to Consider

1. Why has progress against AIDS been spectacular?
2. What is the HTLV-III virus?
3. What treatments have been tried for the AIDS disease?

Excerpted from testimony by James O. Mason before the Subcommittee on Government Operations, February 21, 1985.

We must continue to keep in perspective the extraordinary achievements that have been made to date.

The rate of scientific progress in research on AIDS has been nothing short of spectacular. Never before in the history of medicine has so much been learned about an entirely new disease in so short a time.

What is generally not appreciated is that this extraordinary rate of progress has only been possible because of the existence, when AIDS was first identified in 1981, of a large body of applicable basic scientific knowledge and of a large cadre of prepared epidemiologists, clinicians, and research scientists whose interests, knowledge, and facilities enabled them to move quickly and productively into studies of this new disease. The first two clusters of patients with symptom complex subsequently identified as AIDS were recognized and studied in New York and California in 1981 by clinical research groups working on immunologic disorders with NIH grant support. These clusters were reported to CDC, which then initiated the program of nationwide AIDS surveillance, using personnel and mechanisms already developed and tested in the surveillance of other conditions.

Studies of the pathophysiology of AIDS and the characterization of the underlying immunologic disturbance—the basis for calling the illness acquired immune deficiency syndrome—depended entirely on earlier work using the monoclonal antibody technology to identify and count T and B lymphocytes in patients' blood and to understand the significance of perturbations in these numbers.

Finally, the research leading up to the discovery and characterization of the causative virus, HTLV-III, would have been impossible in the absence of foregoing work on other animal and human retroviruses which were objects of intense interest because of their known or suspected roles in the causation of cancer.

All of this scientific readiness owes its existence to previous decades of strong national support of basic and applied research, epidemiology, and surveillance. Our accomplishments in AIDS are an illustration of that continuing support.

It is interesting to speculate what might have happened if the AIDS epidemic had broken out in 1961 instead of 1981. Lacking most of the scientific tools on which seminal advances have depended, researchers of that day would probably not be beyond clinical and epidemiological descriptions within 3 years.

In fact, the basic unity of the syndrome manifested in some patients by Kaposi's sarcoma and in others by opportunistic infections might not be recognized. It illustrates the wisdom of Pasteur's oft-quoted saying, "Chance favors the prepared mind."

I am here today with my colleagues to address the technical memorandum prepared at your request by the Office of Technology Assessment, titled "Review of the Public Health Service's Response to AIDS". . . .

OTA Report

The OTA report is critical of the administration for increasing AIDS activities through a reallocation of priorities and failing to request budget supplementals and budget amendments. The OTA report asserts that the coordination of PHS resources could be improved. We believe the approach that PHS has taken on reallocating resources was appropriate. We believe it is inherently responsible to shift resources to high priority projects such as AIDS.

As the OTA report notes, over $3 million was shifted into the final fiscal year 1984 AIDS funding plan because the PHS perceived the need for such additional funding. I believe the PHS must be prepared to meet such high priority challenges.

For example, over the past few years the CDC has been responsible for shifting its priorities and resources to meet high priority public health emergencies such as Three Mile Island, Mount St. Helens, Toxic Shock Syndrome, and Legionnaires' disease.

Except for a small increase for Mount St. Helens, the CDC was not provided additional funds for any of these activities. NIH and FDA also have reallocated resources and must continue to be able to reallocate resources to high priority projects.

As with any relatively new and complex public program, the development of firm resource estimates 9 to 12 months in advance of use is difficult. Because of the dynamic nature of the AIDS effort—discovery of causative agent, development of blood test, work toward development of vaccine, preparation of control strategy, et cetera—the development of resource estimates has been difficult. However, this difficulty has not in any way diminished our ability to manage and coordinate the use of our resources to maximize our opportunity to fund the highest priority activities.

In fiscal year 1985 the PHS planned to obligate $96 million for AIDS activities. This represents an increase of $35 million over the fiscal year 1984 level and $64 million over the fiscal year 1983 level. We agree with the OTA report, which describes fiscal year 1984 and fiscal year 1985 funding levels as substantial. For fiscal year 1986, the PHS planned to maintain the fiscal year 1985 operating level of $86 million. The $10 million decrease from fiscal year 1985 is because of one-time fiscal year 1985 expenditures for facility renovations, expansions and blood supply studies.

The fiscal year 1985 and fiscal year 1986 estimates represented the Public Health Service's best estimate of the requirements necessary to continue its efforts to fully understand and ultimately prevent this devastating disease. We will revise these estimates as the need changes.

In summary, my colleagues and I will continue to study the OTA report, searching for possible ways to improve our future efforts in solving the problems of AIDS. We are proud of this Nation's accomplishments to date, but the AIDS battle is not over. It has only just begun. We are ever mindful of the need to pursue the complex questions still before us.

Achievements

We must continue to keep in perspective the extraordinary achievements that have been made to date. Compared to our experiences with another relatively recently recognized viral disease, hepatitis B, much has been accomplished with acquired immune deficiency syndrome in a very short time.

Less than 3 years will have elapsed between the recognition of AIDS as a probable viral disease and the availability of highly sensitive tests for antibody. Achieving the same level of test development for hepatitis B required more than 15 years.

Within the same short period of 3 years, epidemiologic evidence of modes of transmission and laboratory information on the virus appear to have made it possible to remove already one group from high risk of exposure to HTLV-III.

Heat treatment of factor VIII has been shown to destroy the AIDS virus. This action, as well as screening donors by laboratory tests, should reduce the hemophilia patient's risk of AIDS transmitted by the very product that is essential for his well being.

We are also highly pleased with the significant accomplishments of blood banks, State and local health departments and community groups in collaborating with us in instituting measures to protect the Nation's blood supply.

We agree with the OTA report that the number of AIDS cases is increasing rapidly and that there is a real possibility that the infection may spread beyond current groups at risk. We are geared up for a prolonged battle against AIDS. Control and prevention strategies based upon epidemiological and laboratory discovery are being formulated. The foundations for implementing these strategies are being developed at the Federal, State and local levels.

THE NATIONAL RESPONSE

MISHANDLING
THE AIDS THREAT

M. Stanton Evans

*M. Stanton Evans is a nationally syndicated columnist and a
prominent national spokesman for conservative domestic
and foreign policy ideas.*

Points to Consider

1. How has the U.S. Public Health Service been slow in
   responding to the AIDS threat?
2. What misguided reassurances have been given to the
   public?
3. What is "casual contact" and what threat does it pose to
   the public?
4. How are the Center for Disease Control guidelines for
   health care workers described?

M. Stanton Evans, "AIDS Horror Story Worsens," *Human Events*,
November 30, 1985, p.7.

The AIDS virus can show up in just about any body fluid imaginable. What does this suggest about common association in the workplace, schoolyard, or other such setting?

Instead of getting better, the public-health horror story involving official handling of AIDS—the killer disease that attacks the immune defenses of the body—keeps getting worse.

Since this affliction is invariably fatal, you might suppose that people entrusted with protecting the public health would take some air-tight measures to guard against it. From the outset, however, the facts of the case have been the opposite. The custodians of our physical well-being have not only been slow in responding to the threat, but have constantly busied themselves with soothing reassurances that turn out to be mistaken.

Early on, for example, health and blood bank officials were assuring us there was minimal danger of AIDS transmission through the blood supply. When people started dying of transfusion AIDS, that assurance was forgotten. Then we were told we couldn't bar homosexual blood donors, even though the disease is correlated with gay sexual practice. Only "promiscuous" homosexuals were barred from giving blood—until the guidelines were quietly changed this fall, to rule out all practicing male homosexuals.

No Danger

The latest official assurance is a report from the Centers for Disease Control of the U.S. Public Health Service, which tells us there is no danger of getting AIDS through "casual contact," and that there is thus no reason to be concerned about catching the disease in the workplace. In addition, we are told that, "because AIDS is not transmitted through preparation or serving food and beverages, these recommendations state that foodservice workers known to be infected with AIDS should not be restricted from work. . . ."

All very reassuring, right? But then we read the fine print of the CDC recommendations, and discover some things that don't fit in with the flat assertion about no danger through

Casual Contact

In testimony before the Republican Study Committee of the House of Representatives on November seventh, a spokesman for the Department of Health and Human Services noted: "The AIDS virus has been isolated from blood, semen, saliva, tears, and urine. Although it is likely to be isolated from other body fluids, secretions, and excretions, epidemiologic evidence has implicated only blood and sexual contact in transmission. We know of no case of AIDS that has been spread by casual contact. . . ."

We have had repeated assurances from medical politicians that it is "highly improbable" that contact with saliva, urine, or tears—such as might occur in a classroom, cafeteria, hospital, dental office, etc.—will transmit AIDS. An assurance by medical politicians that something is "highly improbable" is just not good enough when we are threatened by an unknown deadly disease and conflicting experts.

Conservative Digest, *December, 1985*

"casual contact," and the lack of concern about AIDS sufferers involved in preparing and handling food. We read, for instance, that the AIDS virus to date "has been isolated from blood, semen, saliva, tears, breast milk, and urine, and is likely to be isolated from some other body fluids, secretions and excretions. . . ."

In other words, the AIDS virus can show up in just about any body fluid imaginable. What does this suggest about common association in the workplace, schoolyard, or other such setting? The spread of contagious diseases in such places, involving close personal contact, sneezing, coughing, handling of common objects, use of common restroom facilities, water fountains and utensils, etc., is well-known. Yet we aren't supposed to worry about such things in the case of AIDS.

The implications in the case of foodhandling are especially chilling. Under these guidelines, an AIDS sufferer could well be preparing or handling the food you eat in a restaurant. Quite apart from the chance of contamination through sneezing, etc., there is the possibility that such a food worker could have a nick or cut that would permit contamination through blood. Nothing to be concerned about, according to our public health officials.

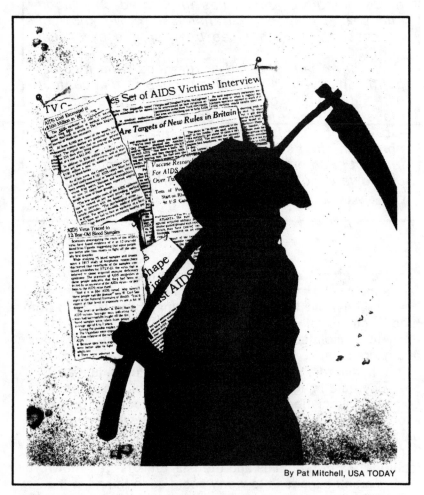

By Pat Mitchell, USA TODAY

The reason for this laid-back approach, we are told, is that so far there have been no known cases of AIDS being transmitted through such contact. Blood and sexual transmission have been the identified culprits to date—not "other body fluids." Therefore, the possibility of getting AIDS in workplaces or restaurants can be discounted. The issue of nicks and cuts is not addressed, though even if it were this new assurance would be less than reassuring.

Guidelines

Reading further in the latest missive from CDC, for instance, we find a series of guidelines for health-care workers to help them avoid catching AIDS from patients. These guidelines state, over and over, that such workers should avoid contact not only with the blood of AIDS patients, but with those "other body fluids" that supposedly aren't a danger to anyone. Here are some representative passages:

"When the possibility of exposure to blood or *other body fluids* exists, routinely recommended precautions should be followed. The anticipated exposure may require gloves alone, as in handling items soiled with blood or equipment contaminated with blood or *other body fluids,* or may also require gowns, masks, and eye coverings when performing procedures involving more extensive contact with blood or *potentially infective body fluids.* . . .

". . .[B]ecause of the *theoretical risk of salivary transmission.* . .during mouth-to-mouth resuscitation, special attention should be given to the use of disposable airway equipment or resuscitation bags and the wearing of gloves when in contact with blood or *other body fluids.* Resuscitation equipment and devices known *or suspected* to be contaminated with blood *or other body fluids* should be used once and disposed of or thoroughly cleaned and disinfected after each use." (Italics added.)

All of this is recommended even though, to date, there has been no known case of health care workers' getting AIDS through "other body fluids." Given the fact that we are still learning about the disease, and that the latency period can last for years, such precautions are obviously quite sensible. We aren't supposed to fret, however, about those other body fluids in the workplace, or in the handling of our food!

PROTECTING THE PUBLIC WELFARE

Public Health Service

The following statement was taken from an AIDS Information Bulletin by the Public Health Service.

Points to Consider

1. What scientific progress has been made against the AIDS virus?
2. What different Public Health Service agencies have been working on a cure for AIDS?
3. What studies are being done by the Center for Disease Control and the National Institute of Health?
4. What national educational program on AIDS prevention was proposed by the Public Health Service?

Excerpted from a Public Health Service Bulletin, November, 1985.

Studies are under way to define further the risk factors for AIDS and to find effective ways to prevent the disease's transmission.

The U.S. Public Health Service (PHS) is working through its health research and surveillance agencies to track the incidence of AIDS, to determine its origin, and to develop effective diagnostic, treatment, and prevention procedures. PHS agencies—the National Institutes of Health (NIH), the Centers for Disease Control (CDC), the Food and Drug Administration (FDA), the Alcohol, Drug Abuse and Mental Health Administration (ADAMHA), and the Health Resources and Services Administration (HRSA)—are carrying out AIDS research and other related activities. . . .

PHS Progress Against AIDS

• A retrovirus, known variously as human T-lymphotropic virus type III (HTLV-III), lymphadenopathy-associated virus (LAV), and AIDS-related virus (ARV), has been identified as the cause of AIDS. In addition, there has been significant progress in describing the structure of the virus and understanding its effect in humans. Infection with the virus does not always lead to AIDS. Preliminary results of studies show that most infected persons remain in good health; others may develop illness ranging in severity from mild to extremely serious.
• In June 1984, PHS licensed five companies to produce a test to identify antibody to the AIDS virus in blood. Less than a year later, the test was in use to screen blood donated for transfusions and for the manufacture of blood products and plasma at the nation's blood centers. The test will be a major factor in reducing still further the number of cases related to blood transfusions or use of blood products.
• More than 100 drugs have been screened to determine their ability to fight AIDS. Other antiviral drugs and drugs to augment the immune system are under study. It is likely that

a combination of the two types of treatments—one to prevent the virus from multiplying in the body, the other to build up the damaged immune system—will be necessary to alter successfully the clinical course of AIDS.

• Studies are under way to define further the risk factors for AIDS and to find effective ways to prevent the disease's transmission. Specific studies include those of (1) risk factors for transmission among 7,000 homosexual men in San Francisco, (2) risk among family members of AIDS patients, (3) AIDS patients reported not to belong to known risk groups, (4) blood donors to patients with transfusion-associated AIDS, (5) risk to health care and laboratory workers from needlestick and mucosal exposures to patients with AIDS, and other related areas.

• A national program to inform the public, high-risk groups, the public health community, and others about AIDS has been under way for 3 years. A national toll-free hotline has responded to nearly 1,000,000 phone calls since July 1983. A summary of activities and accomplishments of the individual agencies of the Public Health Service follows:

Centers For Disease Control: Accomplishments

• Funded cooperative agreements with states and municipalities to carry out active surveillance for AIDS. Assigned public health advisors to high priority areas: New York City, Miami, San Francisco, and Los Angeles. These activities helped establish the national scope of the AIDS epidemic.

• Conducted more than 80 workshops about the use, and supportive counseling related to the use, of the HTLV-III antibody test, for state and local health officers who work with AIDS patients, high-risk group members, and others taking the antibody test at sites other than blood collection agencies.

• Funded and provided technical assistance to the U.S. Conference of Mayors' national AIDS information interchange system among city governments. The exchange program makes timely and appropriate information about AIDS available to mayors and local health officials, especially in high-impact cities.

• Developed a description and definition of AIDS among children.

64

More Funding for Education

Prevention through education on ways of minimizing exposure to HTLV-III has the greatest potential of limiting the spread of AIDS. So far, efforts to prevent AIDS through education have received minimal funding, especially efforts targeted at the groups at highest risk.

Office of Technology Assessment, February, 1985

• Collaborated with the National Institutes of Health in developing an active surveillance system for AIDS in Zaire and in conducting related epidemiologic studies in that country.
• Analyzed surveillance data to provide accurate information on AIDS trends and patterns and to detect any newly emerging risk groups.
• Provides a national toll-free AIDS hotline to supply up-to-date information to the public.

National Institutes of Health

NIH is conducting and supporting multidisciplinary studies aimed at understanding the natural history of AIDS, characterizing the virus that causes the disease, delineating the nature of the immune deficiency in AIDS patients, developing treatments for the opportunistic diseases of AIDS patients, and developing a vaccine in an appropriate animal model.

NIH components undertaking AIDS research include the National Cancer Institute (NCI), the National Heart, Lung and Blood Institute (NHLBI), the National Institute of Allergy and Infectious Diseases (NIAID), the National Institute of Neurological and Communicative Disorders and Stroke (NINCDS), the National Institute of Dental Research (NIDR), the National Eye Institute (NEI), and the Division of Research Resources (DRR).

With NIH support through project grants, contracts, and cooperative agreements, research institutions across the country are also conducting investigations on all aspects of AIDS.

Accomplishments

• HTLV-III, the virus believed to be responsible for causing AIDS, was isolated in 1984 by scientists of the National Cancer Institute. Since that time, these investigators, in collaboration with other NIH researchers and scientists at institutions outside NIH, have mapped the entire genetic structure of HTLV-III and have isolated the virus in blood, semen, saliva, tears, and urine.

• Neurologists at NINCDS have found that nearly half of AIDS patients have neurological complications caused by such problems as opportunistic infections, rare complications of the brain, and subacute encephalitis.

• Investigators at NIH are conducting experimental phase I trials in AIDS patients, using a variety of therapies aimed at reversing the immune defect, destroying the virus, and treating opportunistic diseases.

Information and Education

The Public Health Service has developed a comprehensive plan to inform the American public about AIDS in order to create general awareness and understanding of the syndrome, the ways it is transmitted, and the relative threat it poses to various population groups and to the public health. The ultimate goal of the public information program is to help prevent and control AIDS.

The nature and effects of AIDS and the public response to both of these make it desirable to target selected information and appropriate messages to several audiences. The public needs to know specifically that AIDS is an infectious, sexually transmitted, blood-borne illness. The fact that both homosexual and heterosexual people may be at risk for AIDS because of sexual exposure is a message of importance to all segments of the public. So, too, is the danger posed by drug injection.

Other messages are being tailored to the following groups: homosexual and bisexual men, users of IV drugs, hemophilia patients and their families, blood donors and recipients, sexual partners of people at high risk for contracting AIDS, heterosexuals with multiple sex partners (including prostitutes), people with AIDS-related symptoms, AIDS patients, and health care workers and others whose jobs bring them in close contact with the above groups.

WHAT IS EDITORIAL BIAS?

This activity may be used as an individualized study guide for students in libraries and resource centers or as a discussion catalyst in small group and classroom discussions.

The capacity to recognize an author's point of view is an essential reading skill. The skill to read with insight and understanding involves the ability to detect different kinds of opinions or bias. Sex bias, race bias, ethnocentric bias, political bias and religious bias are five basic kinds of opinions expressed in editorials and all literature that attempts to persuade. They are briefly defined in the glossary below.

5 Kinds of Editorial Opinion or Bias

sex bias— *the expression of dislike for and/or feeling of superiority over the opposite sex or a particular sexual minority*

race bias— *the expression of dislike for and/or feeling of superiority over a racial group*

ethnocentric bias— the expression of a belief that one's own group, race, religion, culture or nation is superior. Ethnocentric persons judge others by their own standards and values.

political bias— the expression of political opinions and attitudes about domestic or foreign affairs

religious bias— the expression of a religious belief or attitude

Guidelines

1. From the readings in chapter two, locate five sentences that provide examples of editorial opinion or bias.

2. Write down each of the above sentences and determine what kind of bias each sentence represents. Is it sex bias, race bias, ethnocentric bias, political bias or religious bias?

3. Make up one sentence statements that would be an example of each of the following: *sex bias, race bias, ethnocentric bias, political bias* and *religious bias.*

4. See if you can locate five sentences that are factual statements from the readings in chapter two.

5. What is the editorial message of the cartoon on page 60?

CHAPTER 3

RELIGIOUS AND MORAL CONFLICTS

RELIGIOUS AND MORAL CONFLICTS

SPIRITUAL SUPPORT NEEDED FOR GAY COMMUNITY

American Lutheran Church

The following comments were excerpted from an eight-page report entitled "AIDS: A Challenge to the Church," which has been sent to American Lutheran congregations in an effort to provide information and stimulate discussion on the disease that could affect—if cases continue to double annually—1 million Americans during the next six years, according to health officials.

The report was developed with information from the U.S. Center for Disease Control in Atlanta, Lutherans Concerned of North America, and a number of AIDS service centers, hospices, chaplains, and doctors.

Points to Consider

1. What does the diagnosis of AIDS mean?
2. How are the challenges to the churches defined?
3. What percent of AIDS cases occur in active homosexual (gay) and bisexual males with multiple partners?
4. How is homophobia described?
5. What specific support can religious organizations give to AIDS patients?

American Lutheran Church, "AIDS: A Challenge to the Church," March 1986, pp. 1-5.

Is it not more than a coincidence that those most devastated by AIDS—gay people, IV drug users, and prostitutes have traditionally been marginalized and abused in our society—and made to feel unwelcome in our churches?

AIDS calls for an enormous amount of sanity, sensitivity, compassion, and level-headedness on behalf of the church and the society at large. It brings us face to face with profound religious questions in regard to sexuality and mortality. Two facts need to be up front in any discussion of the AIDS pandemic. First is that 73 percent of AIDS cases to date have occurred in sexually active homosexual (gay) and bisexual males with multiple partners. The second, that the diagnosis of AIDS means death. . . .

The challenge to the church might be defined as follows:
1. To get past the debate about how God views homosexuality.
2. To help the church and society understand that gay and lesbian people are worth caring for.
3. To demonstrate to gay and lesbian people that they are loved.
4. To get accurate and up-to-date information out to the public.
5. To make public discussion happen that faces up to the political, social, economic, health, religious, and ethical issues at every level of human interaction including the church, school, and government.
6. To carry out a compassionate and caring ministry to those whose lives have been, are, and will be affected by AIDS.
7. To grow in its understanding of who is included in the body of Christ.
8. To live out of the resources of faith rather than to live fearfully.

Human Sexuality

AIDS is a lethal disease. It brings those who are so afflicted face to face with the ultimate reality of death. All of the emotion of denial, anger, and fear are present, but there

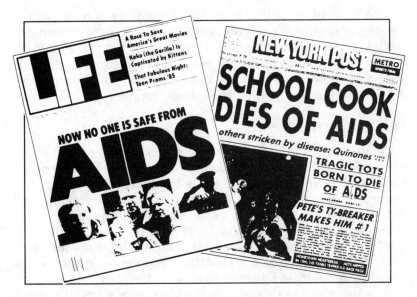

These are some of the more lurid headlines being used by the media. *(The Militant)*

is more. The emotional and spiritual needs of AIDS victims and their families are unusually pressing.

The United States Center for Disease Control (CDC-Atlanta) reports that 73 percent of all AIDS cases are contracted by homosexual or bisexual males. Some people with AIDS had not discussed their sexuality with their families before becoming ill. Think of the trauma parents experience when they are told their son, in the prime of life, has a terminal disease, and then also come to realize that he is gay. AIDS victims and their families in such instances feel the added burden of shame and guilt brought about by the traditional societal and church attitudes toward homosexual people. This often results in alienation from the wider circle of friends and family and they become the outcasts of society. As someone has described it, "As the modern version of the lepers in the days of Jesus."

Congregations should consider the value of studying information about human sexuality in general and homosexuality in particular as part of their ongoing educational and social ministry programs. Pastors and congregational leaders should keep in mind that the typical congregation has a number of homosexual members who may not be known or "visible" to other members. Education can help all members of the congregation be better prepared to assist people with AIDS and their families when a need arises, whether inside the congregation or within the larger communty.

Spiritual Support

It is here the congregation through its members and its pastoral ministry can offer reconciliation, support, and consolation. The spiritual needs for faith, hope, forgiveness, reconciliation, human care and **nonjudgmental** unconditional love are present. Lutherans especially should be familiar with the healing power of grace. There is a place for the public witness that stands against bigotry, indifference, and contempt toward people with AIDS. There is need for the expression and witness for the reverence for life by helping in every way possible to assist individuals with AIDS to live life as comfortably and fully as possible. This includes provision of support and prayer that continues beyond death into the bereavement period for family and loved ones.

AIDS is a syndrome of separation and alienation between the person with AIDS and every support system around him or her. The Christian faith exhorts us to bring salvation (salve) to the brokenness and separation of life.

For the pastoral care provider, the response to people with AIDS should be the same response as to anyone in pain and distress from serious or terminal illness. Since the majority of the patients with AIDS have thus far been homosexual (gay) males, clergy and church people must come to terms with both the diseases of AIDS and HOMOPHOBIA; that is, fear, distress, and hostility toward gay and lesbian people.

God's Wrath

Some well-meaning Christians have raised the question: "Is AIDS God's wrath on homosexuals?" One might respond: "Only if every occurrence of cancer, diabetes, heart disease, or other diseases people suffer are signs of God's wrath as well."

It is not our purpose in this report to discuss the question of whether God approves or disapproves of homosexuality.

74

AIDS and the Ministry

AIDS raises basic issues of pastoral and prophetic ministry that involve the church's role in the community as well as its responsibility for society's dispossessed. Whether or not the federal government or other agencies provide resources to meet this crisis and some of the needs of people touched by it, the church itself must respond if it is to reflect in its life the spirit of its Lord who commanded his fellow servants to do for one another what he had done for them.

The Christian Century, *September 11-18, 1985*

Either way, it does not change the fact that God does not punish through disease. God's love and grace is total and unconditional far beyond our understanding. God does not punish through disease and suffering. God loves us through one another even though disease and suffering happen in our lives. It is through love and caring that people with AIDS and their loved ones will experience life more fully. The AIDS crisis calls us to learn that unconditional love is not a luxury but a basic need of the human condition. Through the example of Job we learn that suffering can come to people in spite of their goodness, and through the teachings of Jesus we learn that the link between sin and disease is broken and the link between forgiveness and love is realized.

Pastors interested in providing ministry to people with AIDS may better serve if they become aware of the various levels of experience gay men and lesbians have had with church or their religious life. Lutherans Concerned, a national organization of homosexual and heterosexual Lutherans concerned for the faith and life issues of gay and lesbians has many chapters located around the country (see resource section) and might well serve in some instances as a contact for a pastoral resource in helping develop such awareness. A number of gay and lesbian people may have completely rejected their religious backgrounds and have had to seek out support and spiritual growth in less traditional ways. It is important that clergy who are neither gay or who have had little or no contact with the gay community take steps to become acquainted with gay people. For example, ministry to the family of an AIDS patient may mean to provide comfort, support, and consultation to a male lover and life partner. People with AIDS are not only faced with the struggle with life-threatening disease to themselves, but many carry the added burden to reach out, support, and educate the significant other people in their lives who also may be dealing with their own distress due to homophobia.

Health Care Workers

Pastors can also support health care workers, including doctors, who face an extremely frustrating series of events—in treating a disease that will not respond. The pastor can help other staff and health care workers cope with their own fears and attitude towards AIDS patients. Pastors can help advocate with community clergy and other church people (home visitors and helpers) that may become involved in behalf of the patient. Pastors and church people can help in intervention, if needed, with social service agencies, funeral homes, home care and nursing homes, who have had a history of refusing care to AIDS patients. Above all, the pastor can bring the traditional prayers, rites, and sacraments of the church which provide strength and a closer union with a God of love and the Christian community that cares. Confession, communion, rites for the sick, Bible study and reflection, preparation for death, funeral services, worship opportunities, and prayer are all gifts of the spirit in love which the pastoral provider can bring. . .

AIDS: A Challenge to the Church

The AIDS crisis challenges the church, and individual Christians, to a deeper and broader self-understanding—to become more fully the community of Christ in the world.

Is it not more than a coincidence that those most devastated by AIDS—gay people, IV drug users, and prostitutes have traditionally been marginalized and abused in our society—and made to feel unwelcome in our churches? How do we grow as an inclusive and open church in the time of AIDS? Are we prepared to embrace people with AIDS, and to respond to their needs as **they** express those needs?

RELIGIOUS AND MORAL CONFLICTS

THE GAY LIFE STYLE MUST BE OPPOSED

Fred Schwarz

Fred Schwarz is the editor and publisher of the Christian Anti-Communism Crusade *newsletter, a conservative publication on moral and political issues.*

Points to Consider

1. How is AIDS transmitted?
2. How serious is the AIDS disease?
3. What different methods can be used to combat AIDS?
4. What is the most effective method?
5. How have attitudes toward homosexuality changed in the past two decades?

Excerpted from three *Christian Anti-Communism Crusade* newsletters, October 15, November 15, and June 1, 1985.

Legislatures, churches, and physicians must combine to protect the community health by stripping the camouflage of legality, morality and normality from this disease-generating life style .

AIDS has triumphed. Rock Hudson is dead. He faced death with courage and dignity. The President and many national personalities have eulogized him on television and radio and in the press.

During his life, his acting gave pleasure to many, and his death was a personal tragedy to the American people. It seems churlish to ask the following question, but it must be faced if we are to prevent the death of future victims of AIDS.

Did he transmit the deadly AIDS virus to others during homosexual contact, thereby causing their death also?

We are informed that Rock Hudson indulged in deviant sexual practices during the latter years of his life. This means he had many partners in homosexual activities. He doubtless had AIDS before he knew he was infectious and possibly transmitted the disease to some of these partners. . . .

The Aids Epidemic

"Acquired Immune Deficiency Syndrome (AIDS) is currently doubling in less-than-a-year intervals and spreading into the heterosexual population—a SWORD OF DAMOCLES of unbelievable proportions."

This alarming statement, which utilizes the symbolism of the ancient myth about the guest who had to sit at the feast with a sword suspended by a single hair above his head, appears in the March 22 edition of the prestigious, authoritative magazine, SCIENCE. This magazine is not noted for panic or overstatement.

The slick left-liberal magazine, MOTHER JONES, which has promoted sexual promiscuity consistently and ardently, is also alarmed. It states: *"The deadly AIDS epidemic has put the entire nation at risk."*

There is just cause for alarm. AIDS is threatening to wipe out a substantial percentage of the U.S. population in the next decade. Let us think the unthinkable and contemplate what the future will bring to pass if the present doubling of the number of victims each year continues:

1985—*8,000 VICTIMS;*   1986—*16,000 VICTIMS;*
1987—*32,000 VICTIMS;*   1988—*64,000 VICTIMS;*
1989—*128,000 VICTIMS;*   1990—*256,000 VICTIMS;*
1991—*512,000 VICTIMS;*   1992—*1,024,000 VICTIMS.*

Continuing this process, almost the entire population of the U.S.A. would be afflicted by the year 2000. AIDS has the destructive potential of the nuclear bomb.

Curbing the Spread of AIDS

This process cannot be allowed to continue. It is not self-terminating, but some procedures are available to halt it. These include:

1. The production of a vaccine which will confer immunity against AIDS:
   There are bright prospects for success in the quest for such a vaccine, but responsible scientists consider that its availability is several years away. The virus associated with AIDS has been isolated, and a test is now available which will reveal with moderate accuracy those people who have antibodies to the AIDS virus in their blood. This is progress, but future developments are hard to predict.

2. The discovery of a medication which will be effective in treating the AIDS disease itself:
   If and when this will come to pass is speculation. However much money is invested in the search, there is no guarantee of success.

3. Prevention of the conduct which promotes the spread of AIDS:
   AIDS originated in association with homosexual promiscuity; it is spreading to the heterosexual population by bisexual promiscuity; and it will spread throughout the heterosexual community by heterosexual promiscuity. Other methods of spreading, such as blood transfusions, are deadly but secondary.

Promiscuity is the primary vehicle for the dissemination of AIDS, and it should therefore be curbed in every way possible. Education and religion have their role to play in this battle, but they should be assisted by appropriate legislation

79

The Principal Carriers

Male homosexuals are the principal victims of AIDS, but they also are the principal carriers of the contagion. This public health problem has been spread throughout our country by an identifiable class of people who engage in a bizarre, risk-taking recreation: frequent promiscuous (often anonymous) homosexual sex.

Phyllis Schlafly, The Independent American, *December, 1985*

which makes promiscuity illegal because of the threat it poses to the health and life of all.

All institutions that promote promiscuity, such as bathhouses and singles bars, should be closed immediately. Conduct likely to spread AIDS should be a crime. . . .

Disease, Sin, Crime

For centuries, homosexual conduct was regarded as a disease by the medical profession, as immoral by religious institutions, and as illegal by government. In the past two decades, this has changed dramatically. The medical profession removed the stigma of disease from homosexual conduct, legislatures removed the stigma of crime, and some religious bodies removed the stigma of sin. The results are now evident. Promiscuity increased exponentially. Investigations have reported that many homosexuals have had more than 500 sexual partners. AIDS now threatens the health and lives of all.

Many excuse homosexual conduct on the grounds that a homosexual has innate urges and preferences over which he has no control. Impulses are one thing; yielding to those impulses is another. Many people are born with a bad temper. This does not excuse their indulgence in acts of violence. They must be taught that violence is wrong and aided in self-control by the knowledge that indulgence will result in legal punishment.

The argument that homosexual conduct between consenting adults hurts only the participants has now lost all validity. Homosexual promiscuity threatens all with AIDS.

80

Legislatures, churches, and physicians must combine to protect the community health by stripping the camouflage of legality, morality and normality from this disease-generating life style. . . .

The Compassionate Treatment of AIDS

Is there any relationship between the AIDS epidemic and the communist strategy to conquer the U.S.A.? There certainly is. The communist formula for conquest is: "External encirclement, plus internal demoralization, plus thermonuclear blackmail, lead to progressive surrender." AIDS is most demoralizing.

While there is agreement that the AIDS epidemic is deadly and increasingly threatens the entire community, there is disagreement concerning what should be done to prevent the spread of the disease. . . .

It is most desirable that medication should be discovered that will cure the disease and a vaccine created which will prevent it, and enormous efforts are being made to achieve these things. There is no guarantee that these efforts will be successful, and the question remains: "What should be done now while the disease is spreading like a prairie fire?" Thousands are dying and millions are threatened while waiting anxiously for the discovery of means to cure or prevent the disease.

The main mechanism by which the disease has been spread is *homosexual conduct.* The second mechanism is intravenous drug use using contaminated needles. The third is the use of infected blood in transfusions.

Education Vs. Legislation

The debate concerns what should be done about the first two of these mechanisms. There are two major schools of thought. These are:
1. Teach people how to engage in homosexual conduct and how to inject drugs without contracting or spreading AIDS.
2. Do everything possible to prevent people from engaging in homosexual conduct and from using drugs.

I read scores of communist and left-wing publications, and their well-nigh universal emphasis is on the former course.

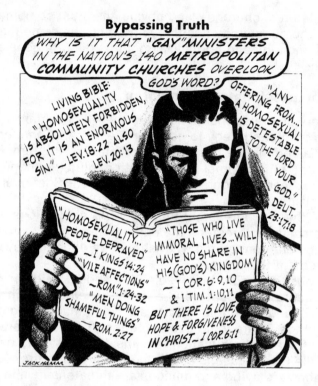

An example is the Sept. 25 to Oct. 1 edition of the Socialist newsweekly, *IN THESE TIMES*. The front page features a graphic presentation of the deadly nature of AIDS picturing an enormous skull with AIDS printed across it in large red letters. Below is the caption: "If present trends continue, AIDS will have killed more Americans by 1988 than died in Vietnam."

The emphasis in the accompanying article is on education as a means of prevention. Testimony given by alleged experts to the Congressional Subcommittee on Intergovernmental Relations and Human Resources, chaired by Rep. Ted Weiss (D.N.Y.), stressed this. The recommended education must teach the practice of "Safe Sex".

One witness protested what he considered to be a barrier to effective education. Jeff Levi, spokesman from the National Gay Task Force (NGTF), said: "How does a public health official support education of gay men about safer sex, in a state that still has sodomy laws on the books, with law enforcement officials still willing to enforce them?"

There we have it. Laws against sodomy hinder the battle against AIDS. The truth is that the abolition of the laws against sodomy has contributed mightily to the spread of AIDS. The abolition of such laws permitted the exponential growth of homosexual conduct—as illustrated by the proliferation of bath houses in San Francisco—and this conduct has had dire results. The radio news to which I listened this morning, quoted the Director of Disease Control in San Francisco, who lamented that over half the *homosexual and bisexual population* of San Francisco are now infected by the AIDS virus and that many will contract the deadly disease itself.

Some "experts" still find it unthinkable that citizens should be hindered by appropriate laws from indulging their impulses, however dangerous such indulgence may be to the entire community. To advocate legal prohibition of homosexual conduct, is to lack compassion. True compassion must consider the plight of thousands who will be affected and infected as a result of such conduct. We already know of heart-rending cases of babies and nuns who have contracted AIDS as a result of receiving blood transfusions from blood that was infected as a result of homosexual conduct.

The obvious lesson is—*homosexual conduct must be minimized by every possible means.* This includes legislation, quarantine, education, social pressure, morality, and spirituality. This is true compassion. . . .

The tragedy is that AIDS continues to be transmitted by homosexual conduct. *If we do not stop homosexual conduct, we will not stop the spread of AIDS.*

Those who support "gay rights" organizations are supporting the death sentence for many who engage in conduct condoned by such rights and possibly for innocent bystanders such as the recipients of blood transfusions and the spouses of bi-sexuals.

Doubtless these truths will offend many, but we are dealing with the issues of life and death, and the truth must be faced so that appropriate measures can be taken to prevent further loss of life.

AIDS IS NOT A GAY DISEASE

Metropolitan Community Church

The following article was prepared as an educational pamphlet by the Metropolitan Community Church in Los Angeles. It was titled "AIDS: Is It God's Judgement?"

Points to Consider

1. Why is AIDS not a punishment from God?
2. Why do people suffer?
3. Is sin punished with disease?
4. Why is AIDS not a gay disease?
5. How is homophobia defined?

Metropolitan Community Church,"AIDS: Is It God's Judgement?"
1985.

If indeed aids is a plague sent by God into the gay community, there are some flaws in the plan. Lesbians are not likely to contract the illness, so then God would not seem to be giving the same sentence to lesbians as to gay men.

Is aids, acquired immune deficiency syndrome, a punishment or scourge from God? Some would say yes. Indeed, some members of what the media calls the religious right would probably praise God for the tragic epidemic which is claiming the lives of thousands of gay men and others. The idea that aids is a punishment from God is based on three false assumptions: That homosexual acts are sinful, that God causes suffering, and that God punishes sin with disease. These false assumptions result from a particular way of looking at society, sexuality, and how God works in the world. These assumptions and the world view they reflect are based on the fear called homophobia, and in tragic misunderstanding of the meaning of Christ. It is the responsibility of Christians to overcome this fear and misunderstanding, and witness to God's love and grace.

Are Homosexual Acts Sinful?

There are a few passages in the Bible that have been said to condemn gay sexual acts. Currently there is much debate about these passages. Some Christians believe these passages condemn *all* homosexual behavior. But a growing number of Bible experts are convinced *these passages condemn only certain sexual acts that are idolatrous or abusive.*

For example, *Sodom and Gomorrah* (Gen. 19), probably deals with rape, which is a violent act and irrelevant to same sex loving relationships. Other passages in the Bible, such as Ezekiel 16:49-50, identify the sin of these cities as injustice and idolatry. Likewise, some religious authorities now point out that New Testament passages like I Corinthians 6:9 and Romans 1:24-27 deal with sexual behavior that is unloving and exploitive (such as prostitution). But even then, the Christian message is one of forgiveness and healing. Jesus said nothing about homosexuality, but he said a

The Church and AIDS

If the churches are to be useful instruments in facing the crisis, they have to examine their theological attitude toward AIDS, seek understanding of the disease, and then move to action, supporting persons with AIDS and efforts to combat the disease.

The first point is theological. The Rev. Jerry Falwell has called AIDS divine retribution on homosexuals. Before he became communications director at the White House, Patrick Buchanan wrote in his syndicated column that homosexuals "have declared war on nature, and now nature is exacting an awful retribution."

Such a position is untenable intellectually and appalling theologically. If God is punishing homosexuals, then why do lesbians not contract AIDS? Why is African experience of AIDS largely heterosexual? If God is engaged in germ warfare against sinners, then why do those whose sins affect many more people more profoundly—drug dealers, slum landlords, polluters, war makers—not receive similar punishments?

Christianity and Crisis, *December 9, 1986*

great deal about faith, hope and love.

Certain passages of the Bible, around which there is no debate, assure us that everyone has access to God by faith. John 3:16 teaches that **whosoever** believes in Christ will have eternal life. Gay persons who believe in Christ are part of the "whosoevers," mentioned in John.

Does God Cause Suffering?

Why do people suffer? All religions have had to address this question. Our world is full of human suffering caused by hunger, disease, poverty and multiple forms of oppression and injustice. If these things are happening, does this mean they are God's will and, therefore, God wills us to suffer?

Evil is a very real force in this world, a force *not* of God's making. (Mark 1:32-34) And aids is certainly a devastating evil not of God's will. It is not "just deserts" for gay men sent them as punishment. Jesus never punished people with sickness. He healed. *Aids is a tragedy, and God suffers with all who are victimized by it or lose loved ones because of it.*

Bad things do happen to good people! We suffer many times through no fault of our own, because the world is many times an unfair, unjust place. God's created order exists among chaos that is not of God.

God does not cause the tragedy but God does respond to suffering with healing. God heals sometimes through physical restoration, at other times with grace sufficient to grow in the midst of suffering. (I Corinthians 12:9)

God's healing is described by a woman with a friend who died of aids: "He was an abused child, abandoned by his mother. But in his last months, his mother came to live with him, nursing him around the clock. In their times together old wounds were healed, forgiveness was shared and faith grew. My friend received a healing gift of family and love he had never known."

Even when the injustice of tragedy invades our lives, God's passionate love can bring good in the form of healing and growth. We can find God's healing touch in our tears of sadness and our screams of anger. We can find God's healing touch in the words of love and comfort shared by others. More than anything, we can find God's healing touch through that inner peace that comes from God's presence and promises. We know that in everything God works for good with those who love God. (Romans 8:28)

Is Sin Punished with Disease?

"Is God punishing Gays with aids?" This is the kind of question that has been asked for centuries, substituting many other names for aids and many other communities for gay. Each time some mysterious malady befalls a nation or an identified community there is the rush to see if God did it and if so, why. If indeed aids is a plague sent by God into the gay community, there are some flaws in the plan. Lesbians are not likely to contract the illness, so then God would not seem to be giving the same sentence to lesbians as to gay men. And, there is the matter of all the other peo-

'We thank thee for the gifts of thy bountiful herpes and thy blessed AIDS, oh Lord . . . now send us something for all the other weirdos.'

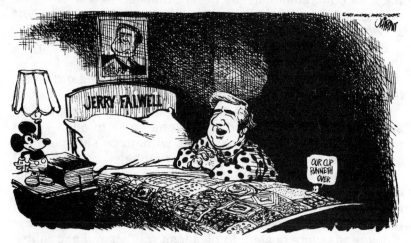

ple who are not gay that are affected. What do we do with all the people in the country of Zaire where there is the highest case rate in the world for aids and it has nothing to do with IV drug use or sexual orientation? Clearly there is no justification for suggesting that God has found disfavor with the gay community (males only), and has created aids as punishment. Are all women with toxic shock syndrome victims of God's wrath? Or Blacks with sickle cell anemia? Or Jews with Tay-Sachs disease?

People had similar questions during the time of Jesus Christ. Then, as now, many assumed that suffering is a direct result of sin. But Christ challenged that assumption.

As Jesus walked along, he saw a man who had been blind from birth. His disciples asked him, "Rabbi, was it his sin or that of his parents that caused him to be blind?" "Neither," answered Jesus, "it was no sin, either of this man or of his parents. Rather it was to let God's work show forth in him." (John 9:1-3)

Jesus then reached out to heal the blind man. We too, must reject the idea that aids, or any other illness, is punishment for sin. We, like Jesus Christ, must reach out with a healing touch. Rather than God's retribution, suffering becomes an occasion for God's love to be demonstrated. *When Christians reach out and touch those with aids, they can transform suffering into a living example of God's love.*

What Is Our Responsibility?

While our culture often focuses on sin and evil as an individual matter, the Bible speaks frequently of sin as something we are involved in together. Evil comes in groups, in structures, in forces beyond the individual, just as aids is beyond the individual. And our response to aids must be a group response as well as an individual one.

If loving homosexual acts are not evil and God does not cause suffering or punish gays with aids, then what keeps our community from responding? One answer is homophobia. Homophobia is an unrealistic fear of and rejection of lesbians and gay men.

Homophobia affects *us* when we believe that there is something wrong with our sexuality. We question the validity of who we are and give in to self-hatred. This is not surprising, since we are taught homophobia from a young age through such things as queer jokes, and a lack of positive role models. Facing that fear is the first step toward ending the paralysis which effects much of our community. As we become more free of homophobia, we can work toward the elimination of this tragic disease.

"The Truth shall set us free," and yet we too often deny the truth or avoid learning about aids because of fear. It is our community responsibility to educate ourselves and all we can reach. Many in our community have fears about the risks of contracting aids; we must overcome our fear with facts.

Like Jesus with the lepers, as a community we are called to **eat** with people with aids and **share** their home with them (Matthew 26:6); **touch** people with aids and **give** them our intimacy (Matthew 8:2-4); and to **heal** people with aids (Luke 17:11-19.) *Our faithful, intimate presence in the lives of those with aids, witnessing to them of Jesus' healing touch, is one of the most important responsibilities we have.*

RELIGIOUS AND MORAL CONFLICTS

GAY EPIDEMIC THREATENS OUR HEALTH

Norman Podhoretz

Norman Podhoretz is the editor of Commentary *magazine and a prominent national spokesman for conservative opinions on domestic and international issues.*

Points to Consider

1. How does the public feel about homosexuality?
2. Why are gay men responsible for spreading the AIDS disease?
3. How could the AIDS disease be stopped without a vaccine or drug?

Reporters have used vague phrases like "exchange of bodily fluids" or "intimate sexual contact," and they have rarely pointed to "the correlation between AIDS and extreme promiscuity."

When AIDS first appeared among us a few years ago, it was, not unreasonably, expected to unleash a wave of revulsion against homosexuality—or "homophobia," as it has come to be derisively called by all who believe that it is this feeling of revulsion, rather than homosexuality itself, which is abnormal or unnatural.

Yet, while there has been a good deal of revulsion felt and expressed in private, the public response has been a meek acceptance of the idea propagated by homosexual activists that it is the rest of us who are responsible for the existence and spread of this horrible disease.

From the idea that the rest of us are to blame, it follows that we must give "top priority" to halting the spread of AIDS. This, in fact, is what the Reagan administration, speaking through the president himself, has agreed to do.

The Implications

There are extraordinary implications here, but before they can be clearly brought out, a little history has to be reviewed.

At first, then, as part of the campaign to saddle the whole of society with the responsibility of AIDS, homosexual activists appealed not only to our compassion but to our self-interest. Unless something was done quickly, they told us, there was a great danger that the disease would spread beyond the homosexual world and into the population at large.

AIDS, in other words, as the executive director of the Gay Men's Health Crisis insisted, was not "merely a disease of a socially disapproved life style," it was everyone's business.

But these warnings of a general epidemic quickly backfired. Instead of creating a sense among heterosexual people of solidarity with homosexuals, they aroused the very revulsion that the activists had been trying to ward off. People began to be afraid of coming into any kind of contact with homosexuals for fear that they might be infected.

Shift in Strategy

At that point, and with panic gathering in the air, the strategy shifted back to an appeal for compassion. At the same time, in conjunction with the debate over allowing children with AIDS into the classroom, the scientific authorities rushed in to assure us that the disease could almost certainly not be caught by casual contact. Furthermore, they added, all the evidence showed that AIDS was still overwhelmingly confined to homosexuals and intravenous-drug users and was not spreading to the population at large.

Now the scientists have gone even further. This month, Dr. James Mason, director of the National Centers for Disease Control in Atlanta, flatly stated that no new drug or vaccine is needed to halt the spread of AIDS. "We could stop transmission of this disease today," he said, if only homosexuals (and intravenous-drug users—but they are another story) were willing to observe certain precautions.

In speaking of these precautions, however, the news media, with one or two exceptions like the New York Post, have, as Newsweek puts it, surrendered to "a squeamish lack of specificity." Reporters have used vague phrases like "exchange of bodily fluids" or "intimate sexual contact," and they have rarely pointed to "the correlation between AIDS and extreme promiscuity."

Gay... the Great Misnomer

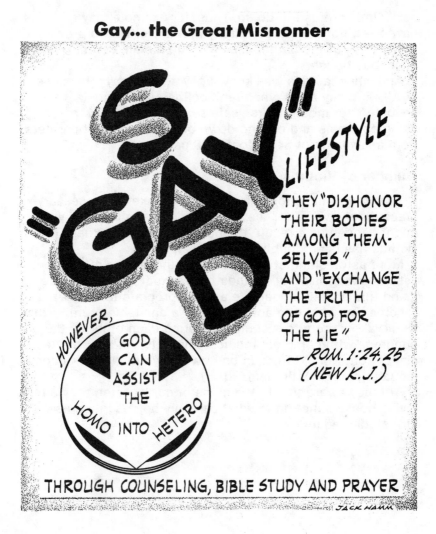

Curious, is it not, that in an age of ubiquitous pornography and blunt speech, it should be so hard to say in plain English that AIDS is almost entirely a disease caught by men who bugger and are buggered by dozens or even hundreds of other men every year?

Yet an amazing proportion of these men who could protect themselves and their "lovers" by giving up such "joys of gay sex" simply refuse to do so. Thus, for example, gay activists have been fighting, successfully in many cities, to prevent the closing of the bathhouses that are a main center of promiscuous buggery.

And while, as one well-known gay activist says, because of AIDS "many of us who aren't celibate are almost celibate," for most others "safe sex" evidently now means using condoms and cutting down on the number of partners from an average of 64 to "only" 18 per year.

Number of Victims

Thanks to this astonishing refusal to take the necessary precautions even after they had every reason to know what might happen as a result, the number of homosexual AIDS victims has been doubling every year.

More astonishing still, not only do these men refuse to assume responsibility for their own sexual habits; they demand that society undertake a crash program to develop a vaccine—or what one activist calls "a one-tablet cure"—that would allow them to resume buggering each other by the hundreds with complete medical impunity. And the politicians, from Ronald Reagan on down, have rushed to accommodate this fantastic demand.

Are they aware that in the name of compassion they are giving social sanction to what can only be described as brutish degradation?

RELIGIOUS AND MORAL CONFLICTS

MORALISTS SHOULD STOP CLOUDING AIDS DEBATE

Allan M. Dershowitz

Alan M. Dershowitz is a professor at the Harvard Law School. He has been a prominent national spokesman on moral and legal issues.

Points to Consider

1. What exaggerated warnings about AIDS have been heard?
2. What scientific facts surprised a Harvard Medical School audience?
3. How do conservative moralists describe the AIDS issue?
4. What do the gay activists say?
5. How can the moralistic debate harm the efforts to learn about AIDS?

Those who have a stake in using AIDS to prove the morality or immorality of any particular life style should be deemed disqualified from scientific debate.

The time has come to take the moralism and politics out of the informational part of the debate over AIDS. Let the moralists and the politicians continue to argue about the social-policy decisions that necessarily have to be made in response to the AIDS epidemic. But *let the flow of scientific information be unpolluted by personal moralism.*

We have all heard exaggerated warnings about AIDS from moral majoritarians who want carriers quarantined, from frightened parents seeking to keep young AIDS victims out of school and from opportunistic politicans capitalizing on a national hysteria over a dreaded disease whose victims are easy targets for condemnation.

Medical Facts

When Prof. William Haseltine of the Harvard Medical School recently gave his university audience some of the scientific facts about AIDS, there was a stunned silence. "Anyone who tells you categorically that AIDS is not contracted by saliva is not telling you the truth." AIDS may, in fact, be transmissible by tears, saliva, bodily fluids and mosquito bites.

"There are sure to be cases," he continued, "of proved transmission through casual contact."

Unlike the conservative moralists who rail about AIDS, Haseltine has no political ax to grind. He is one of the most prominent scientific leaders in AIDS research, part of a team that has already made some important breakthroughs in identifying the reproductive mechanisms of the AIDS virus.

He—along with a growing number of medical experts—is concerned that the small amount of scientific light that can now be shed in the AIDS controversy is being distorted by enormous quantities of moralistic heat.

Conservative Moralists

Since AIDS is transmitted largely by homosexual conduct and intravenous heroin use, the disease has provided a field day for conservative moralists. Patrick Buchanan, the White House aide and former syndicated columnist, shed crocodile tears over the "poor homosexuals (who) have declared war on nature and now nature is extracting an awful retribution."

Norman Podhoretz, editor of Commentary, has condemned concerned politicians "from Ronald Reagan on down" for undertaking a crash program to develop a vaccine: "Are they aware that in the name of compassion they are giving social sanction to what can only be described as brutish degradation?"

There is an almost gleeful nastiness to the "I-told-you-so" gloating of some conservative moralists who see AIDS as a naturalistic confirmation of the immorality of homosexuality.

On the other side, some gay activists see the public response to AIDS as a political confirmation of society's homophobia.

They refuse to acknowledge that some of the responsibility for the transmission of the disease falls squarely on those homosexuals who have persisted in irresponsible sexual practices even after the dangers became clear.

The movement to keep open "high risk" sex emporiums—bath houses and other establishments where on-premises anal and oral sex is encouraged—plays right into the hands of the conservative moralists.

A representative of the Coalition of Lesbian and Gay Rights charges that guidelines for shutting down high-risk sex hangouts "are a publicity stunt designed to take the heat off the state and put it on gay men." She claims that the guidelines "ignore everything we know about AIDS."

The quest for scientific enlightenment in the battle against AIDS has been hampered by the unfortunate reality that the disease is transmitted by morally controversial practice.

The Moral Debate

Scientists must not be influenced by the moralistic debate. They should consider the disease as if it were transmitted by neutral conduct—in the way that polio was

2 Million People Exposed

Some states, notably California and Wisconsin, have passed laws that ban the use of testing as a barrier to employment or health insurance. But a huge employer, the military, is setting a precedent for other employers and health insurers. If the military can do it, so can the factory.

In the end, the mass-screening program may itself become a public-health danger. It turns attention from finding medical answers to finding social solutions. It feeds the illusion that we can segregate all the people who have been exposed to the virus. But there are an estimated 2 million such people. Until we find a medical cure, they and their problems will touch us every day.

Ellen Goodman, The Boston Globe, *January 14, 1986*

believed, when I was a child, to be caused by swimming in cold water.

Those who have a stake in using AIDS to prove the morality or immorality of any particular life style should be deemed disqualified from the scientific debate.

If the issue were whether a particular disease was caused by eating pork, we surely would not want the scientific arbiters to include Orthodox rabbis or fundamentalist mullahs who might have a stake in proving the wisdom of religious prohibitions.

We have a right to know the hard facts about AIDS, unvarnished by moralistic prejudgments from either side. We also have the right to hear the painful truth from our government agencies, such as the Centers of Disease Control.

AIDS Hysteria

Understandably, such agencies see their role as informing without alarming. But AIDS hysteria—what some people are calling "Afr-AIDS"—should not be allowed to serve as an excuse for understating the problem.

As one distinguished university scientist put it: "We outside the government are freer to speak" than are the Centers for Disease Control, and the "fact is that the dire predictions of those who have cried doom ever since AIDS appeared haven't been far off the mark."

Haseltine has warned: "If you think you're tired of hearing about AIDS now, I can tell you we're only at the beginning."

Let's start hearing more objective information so that each of us can apply our own morality to the difficult social-policy choices we will face as the AIDS epidemic spreads.

RECOGNIZING AUTHOR'S POINT OF VIEW

This activity may be used as an individualized study guide for students in libraries and resource centers or as a discussion catalyst in small group and classroom discussions.

Many readers are unaware that written material usually expresses an opinion or bias. The capacity to recognize an author's point of view is an essential reading skill. The skill to read with insight and understanding involves the ability to detect different kinds of opinions or bias. Sex bias, race bias, ethnocentric bias, political bias and religious bias are five basic kinds of opinions expressed in editorials and all literature that attempts to persuade. They are briefly defined in the glossary below.

5 Kinds of Editorial Opinion or Bias

sex bias—   *the expression of dislike for and/or feeling of superiority over the opposite sex or a particular sexual minority*

race bias—   *the expression of dislike for and/or feeling of superiority over a racial group*

ethnocentric bias—the expression of a belief that one's own group, race, religion, culture or nation is superior. Ethnocentric persons judge others by their own standards and values.

political bias—the expression of political opinions and attitudes about domestic or foreign affairs

religious bias—the expression of a religious belief or attitude

Guidelines

1. Summarize the author's point of view in one sentence for each of the following opinions:

Reading 11 _____

_____

_____

Reading 12 _____

_____

_____

Reading 13 _____

_____

_____

Reading 14 _____

_____

_____

Reading 15 _____

_____

_____

2. Determine what kind of bias each sentence represents. Is it **sex bias, race bias, ethnocentric bias, political or religious bias?**

3. Make up one sentence statements that would be an example of each of the following: **sex bias, race bias, ethnocentric bias, political bias** and **religious bias.**

CHAPTER 4

THE POLITICS OF AIDS

SOCIETY MUST DISCRIMINATE

Richard Restak

Richard Restak is an author and neurologist who has been studying AIDS as a brain related disease.

Points to Consider

1. Why should society identify with the "common good" and not the AIDS victim?
2. In some quarters, how is society responding to the AIDS disease?
3. Why should quarantines for AIDS victims be considered?
4. Why is AIDS not a civil rights issue?

Richard Restak, "When A Plague Looms, Society Must Discriminate", *The Washington Post,* September, 1985. Reprinted with permission.

The benefit of the doubt should not be given to the victim of AIDS. This is not a civil rights issue.

Paradoxically, the truly humanitarian position in the face of an AIDS plague is that we not identify with the victims and instead cast our lot with what in earlier times was dubbed the "common good."

More than 1 million Americans may have been infected with the AIDS virus. And the 13,000 Americans with confirmed cases of the disease, whose number is doubling every year, should be treated with the care and compassion due to anyone who is ill with a so-far incurable and invariably fatal disease. This shouldn't be confused, however, with a refusal to make painful, sometimes anguishing but nonetheless necessary distinctions in the interest of diminishing the likelihood that this awful disease will spread further.

Plagues are not new. They have been encountered in every age and among every nationality: syphilis among the Spanish, bubonic plague among the French, tuberculosis among the Eskimos, polio among Americans.

A New Response

What is new are efforts by medically unsophisticated politicians and attorneys to dictate policy in regard to an illness that has the potential for wreaking a devastation such as has not been encountered on this planet in hundreds of years.

Also different is the response that, in some quarters, is being suggested: Accept the AIDS victim into our schools, place little or no restrictions on employment or housing. The AIDS victims' "rights" in these areas, we are told, should take precedence over the incompletely determined potential for these victims to spread this dread illness.

What some are describing as "discrimination" and "segregation" has a long history in medicine. Quarantines have been effective in beating outbreaks of scarlet fever, smallpox and typhoid in this century. Indeed, by protecting the healthy from the ill we follow a long-established, sensible and ultimately compassionate course. Throughout history true humanitarianism has traditionally involved the compassionate but firm segregation of those afflicted with communicable diseases. Through such a policy diseases have been contained.

Only sentimentalists refuse to make any distinction between the victims of a scourge and those not yet afflicted. Scientists still are unsure why the AIDS virus targets the white blood cells that are the one indispensable element of the body's immune system. But the threat of AIDS demands from us all a discrimination based on our instinct for survival against a peril that, if not controlled, can destroy this society. This is a discrimination that recognizes that caution is in order when knowledge is incomplete. This argument is not a counsel against good medical care or proper concern for AIDS victims. Nor is it a suggestion that we curtail any "civil right" that doesn't potentially imperil the lives of others.

Civil Rights

The humanitarian response to AIDS is exactly the opposite of a humanitarian response to sexism or racism: In the presence of considerable ignorance about the causes and effects of the syndrome, the benefit of the doubt should not be given to the victim of AIDS. This is not a civil-rights issue; it is a medical issue. To take a position that the AIDS virus must be eradicated is not to make judgments on morals or life styles. It is to say that the AIDS virus has no civil rights.

On Aug. 14 the Los Angeles City Council unanimously approved an ordinance making it illegal to discriminate against AIDS patients in regard to jobs, housing and health care. "We have an opportunity to set an example for the whole nation, to protect those people who suffer from AIDS against insidious discrimination," said the councilman who introduced the measure . . . .

Councilman Ernani Bernardi said the ordinance was meant to educate the public to "prevent hysteria."

Preventing hysteria is good. But doctors have not yet made up their minds on the degree of contact required for the disease to be spread from one person to another.

Consider, for example, the varied and patently contradictory measures put into effect across the country in response to the recent discovery that the AIDS virus can be isolated from a victims's tears.

At Boston University, when an AIDS patient is examined, "We are not using the applanation tonometer (a device that tests for glaucoma) because we don't feel we can adequately sterilize it," said the chairman of the department of ophthalmology.

The Massachusetts Eye and Ear Infirmary specialists plan to "review our technique." Translation: We're not sure yet what we're going to do.

In San Francisco, the chief of the eye service routinely sterilizes his optic instruments with merthiolate, which "as far as I know" kills the AIDS virus.

The AIDS virus has been isolated from blood, semen, serum, saliva, urine and tears. If the virus exists in these fluids, wisdom dictates that we assume it can also be transmitted by these routes.

It seems reasonable, therefore, that AIDS victims should not donate blood or blood products, should not contribute to semen banks, should not donate tissues or organs to organ banks, should not work as dental or medical technicians and probably should not be employed as food handlers.

While the Los Angeles ordinance exempts blood banks and sperm banks, it's prepared to exert the full power of the law against nonconformists who exclude AIDS sufferers from employment in restaurants, hotels, barber shops and dental offices.

According to the new law, then, a person afflicted with AIDS may, if he is properly trained, work as a dental hygienist. He may clean your teeth. He may clean your teeth even if he has a paper cut on one of his fingers of which he is barely aware. . . .

CDC spokesmen and other AIDS authorities, including Dr. Arye Rubenstein, who treats the largest group of children with AIDS, may be correct in stating that there is "overwhelming evidence that AIDS is not a highly contagious disease." However, in a combined interview, they gave the following responses to an interviewer's questions:

Q. Suppose my child got into a fight with an AIDS victim and both began to bleed?

A. That kind of fight with a possible exchange of body fluids would arouse some concern about transmission of the virus.

Q. What if my child is in a classroom with an AIDS victim who threw up or had diarrhea?

A. Such events would be a matter of concern. In its guidelines, the CDC said that AIDS victims who cannot control body secretions should be kept out of ordinary classrooms.

Q. Suppose a child with AIDS bit my child?

A. Again, a bite would arouse concern.

Any grade-school teacher can attest that "body-fluid contamination" in the form of scratching, throwing up, diarrhea, biting and spitting are everyday fare within a normal schoolroom. That's why infectious diseases like the flu spread through schools like flash fires. It is difficult to imagine how the CDC or anyone else is going to make individual determinations under such circumstances.

What if future research shows that AIDS can be caught in ways other than those already identified? Isn't it more sensible to forgo premature steps against "discrimination" and await scientific developments?

A True Plague

AIDS is not about civil rights, political power or "alternative life styles." It's a disease, a true plague that already, in the words of infectious-disease expert Dr. John Seale, writing in the August issue of Britain's Journal of the Royal Society of Medicine, is capable of producing "a lethal pandemic throughout the crowded cities and villages of the Third World of a magnitude unparalleled in human history."

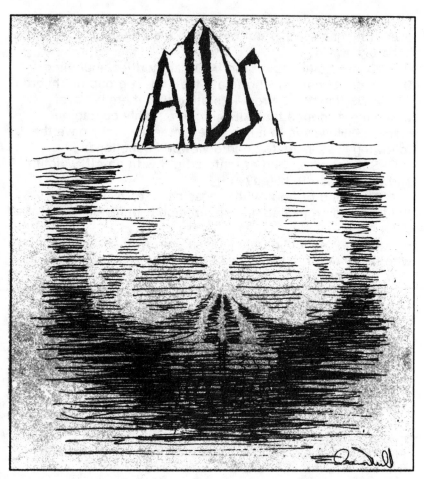

Eleanor Mill sketch

Further, this disease is only partially understood, is untreatable, and is invariably fatal. For these reasons alone, caution would seem to be in order when it comes to exposing the public to those suffering from this illness.

But in addition, the incubation period is sufficiently lengthy to cast doubt on any proclamations, no matter how seemingly authoritative, in regard to the transmissibility of the illness: "The virus may be transmitted from an infected person many years before the onset of clinical manifestations," according to Dr. George Lundberg, editor of the Journal of the American Medical Association. "Latency of many years may occur between transmission, infection and clinically manifest disease."

Truly authoritative statements regarding AIDS cannnot be made. "The eventual mortality following infection. . .cannot be ascertained by direct observation till those recently infected have been followed well into the 21st century," according to Seale.

Given these realities, lawyers and legislators should ponder long and hard whether they wish, by means of legal maneuvering, to create situations—child AIDS victims in the schools, adult AIDS victims working in medical or dental offices and other health-care facilities—in which those afflicted are in a position to pass this virus on to the general public.

The most pressing issue is to arrive at an understanding of all of the ways in which the AIDS virus spreads. But until we do that, political posturing, sloganeering, hollow reassurances and the inappropriate application of legal remedies to a medical problem can only make matters worse and potentially imperil us all.

POLITICS OF AIDS

BLAMING THE VICTIM

James B. Nelson

James B. Nelson is professor of Christian ethics at United Theological Seminary of the Twin Cities of Minneapolis and St. Paul, Minnesota, and author of Human Medicine *(Augsburg, 1984) and* Between Two Gardens: Reflections on Sexuality and Religious Experience *(Pilgrim, 1983). His "Homosexuality and the Church" (Christianity and Crisis, April 4, 1977) is a widely quoted and reprinted contribution to religious understanding of homosexuality.*

Points to Consider

1. Why is hysteria over the casual transmission of AIDS groundless?
2. Why is AIDS not a "gay disease?"
3. What individual rights are at stake in the AIDS controversy?
4. What five guidelines should public policy makers follow in controversy concerning AIDS?
5. How have churches responded?

James B. Nelson, "Responding to, Learning From AIDS", *Christianity and Crisis,* May 19, 1986, pp. 176-81. Reprinted with permission.

AIDS has become one of history's classic examples of "blaming the victim."

It is increasingly clear that this is an epidemic of extraordinarily serious proportions. If the rate of *infection* has slowed slightly in some areas, the dramatic increases in actual *cases* of AIDS will certainly continue for the foreseeable future. The number of persons in high risk groups exposed to the virus, more over, has increased dramatically. (In San Francisco, the 1980 estimate for gay and bisexual males exposed to the AIDS virus [HTLV-III] was 8 percent; in 1986 the estimate is 80 percent.) In spite of occasional hopeful reports, it is unrealistic to expect either a vaccine or a cure in the near future. Thus, the main hope for containing the epidemic in the next several years will continue to lie mainly in the screening of all donated blood, and in education toward modifying high-risk sexual practices and intravenous drug abuse.

We now know that the hysteria over casual transmission has been virtually groundless. Overwhelming data now make it clear that the chances for contracting the virus through nonsexual contact is almost negligible. According to Dr. Merle A. Sande, a leading AIDS specialist at San Francisco General Hospital, writing in the February 6 *New England Journal of Medicine,* "It is now time for members of the medical profession, armed with this knowledge, to take a more active and influential role in quelling the hysteria over casual transmission of AIDS. We need to support public and medical officials who oppose universal screening, quarantine, the exclusion of students from classrooms, and the removal of employees, including health care workers, from the work place."

The hysteria continues, nevertheless. In AIDS, the fears which surround those two most anxiety-ridden dimensions of human life—sexuality and death—powerfully join together. Add to this the irrational fear of homosexuality in a particularly homophobic society, and there is the prescription for trouble.

111

One of the puzzling and difficult things about the present epidemic is the conjunction of two facts: (1) AIDS as such is *not* "a gay disease"; (2) however, in the U.S. it is strongly associated with gay and bisexual males. (National figures indicate 73 percent; when the New York-Newark area—where high drug incidence accounts for more than half of the cases—is removed from the statistical summary, gay and bisexual males constitute something over 90 percent of the AIDS cases nationally.) And the epidemic crisis—of which, tragically, we are seeing only the beginning—is enormously complicated and magnified by homophobia. White racism is a serious companion complication, given the Haitian/African AIDS connections and the fact that intravenous drug abusers involve a disproportionate number of people of color. The focus of this article on homophobia should in no way blind us to the racism issue.

AIDS has become one of history's classic examples of "blaming the victim." The logic seems to go like this: Homosexuality is a freely chosen orientation; because it is both immoral and an illness, one illness leads to another. Further, the logic suggests, since sexual orientation is a perfectly appropriate way of categorizing the essence of human beings, it is perfectly appropriate to treat AIDS as "a homosexual disease"—in spite of the fact that there are no "heterosexual diseases." Thus, a medical diagnosis becomes a moral diagnosis, and vice versa. . . .

Public and Private Rights

In certain ways, the public policy issues now surrounding AIDS seem, on the surface, to be a classic case of individual rights versus the social good. The individual rights at stake are at least of two major types: the right to adequate health care and the right to privacy. Both have been widely affirmed, if not always honored in practice, for all members of our society.

The right to adequate health care for persons with AIDS has been seriously compromised by the slowness of response by many in medicine and government. It is difficult to avoid the conclusion that those at high risk for AIDS did not seem as significant as the populations affected by previous epidemics. Even as medicine has gradually mobilized to cope with this disease, adequate health care in many

AIDS in Prison

Near panic and lack of knowledgeable leadership characterize the situation in prisons across the country, where the problem of inmates with AIDS is growing rapidly.

The same public misconceptions which have led to school boycotts and calls for quarantines are affecting the behavior of those most directly involved: guards and inmates. In several upstate New York prisons, inmates with AIDS have been placed in isolation, often in cells designed for disciplinary purposes. Inmates have been denied access to physical and educational programs solely because they have AIDS.

Jeff Jones, The Guardian, *December 4, 1985*

hospitals is still compromised by fearful staff members who distance themselves from AIDS patients in a variety of ways—in spite of the scientific evidence against casual transmission.

Still another right-to-care issue looms ahead of us. In a society which largely blames the victim for having this disease, will resource allocation for patient care be adequate as numbers and costs dramatically mount?

In ethics and public policy generally, considerations of social good are always relevant and important. Sometimes the social good does indeed demand that individual rights be modified or even curtailed. But those cases should always demand special care and justification. Such has not been the case in regard to persons with AIDS. It is difficult to argue that the nature of medicine's response to AIDS has been justified because large numbers of others have higher health priorities. Likewise, it is difficult to argue that the withdrawal of hospital personnel from patients with AIDS can be justified by the social good of larger numbers of other patients.

The right to privacy shows a similar story. One instance of this right is that of sexual expression between consenting adults. Regarding gays, this right is legally established in only some jurisdictions. The presence of sodomy statutes and the absence of effective civil rights laws in many other areas testifies to the spottiness of legal protection. In any event, the closing of gay bathhouses in certain cities raises a troublesome and rather complex issue of privacy rights. Though bathhouses are patronized by only a minority of the gay population, their closing represents questionable discrimination against persons who have already borne an undue burden of social prejudice. Empirically, there is evidence that sexual activity in many bathhouses has changed to lower-risk expressions and that frequently these establishments have functioned as educational sites for safer sex practices. Thus, the positive results of these closings are not unambiguously clear. Quite possibly, shutting them may even be counterproductive, not only removing locations for safer sex education for some of the most high risk persons of the high risk group, but also contributing to a climate of alienation which inhibits cooperation with public health efforts. The bathhouse closings frequently have been portrayed as obviously justified by the wider social good. But the case is more complex than that.

Another challenge to privacy rights, potentially much more far-reaching in its impact, is the issue of confidentiality. Who has the right to the names of those who receive an HTLV-III positive blood test? Only the affected individuals? Their sex partners? Employers? Insurance companies? Offices of the city, state, and federal government? The military? It is important to remember that a positive blood test only means *exposure* to the HTLV-III virus. It does not indicate that the individual has or will ever get AIDS. It is also no secret that many groups seriously want possession of this information. Some have already pressed blood-testing centers for such data. When an insurance company argues its right to know on grounds of its own financial self-interest, for example, that argument is still predictably clothed in language of the common good.

If we start from the other end, the social good, important considerations also arise. The health of the whole is a legitimate concern of any society. Thus, questions of mass

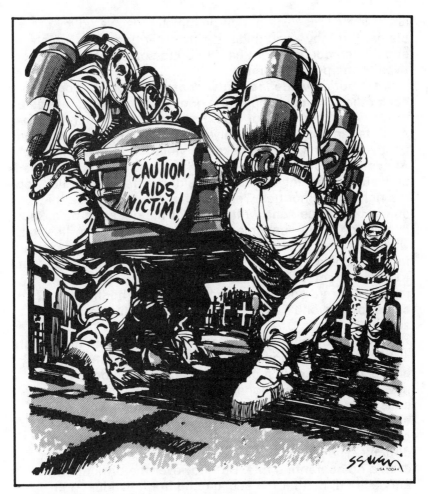

screening, of protecting the blood supply, of protecting health care personnel, of notifying recipients of blood from donors now found to have the virus, of protecting school children, of allocating medical resources in the face of draining expenditures—all are legitimate issues, though in the AIDS crisis they have frequently been compounded by ignorance and fear.

Are there any procedural principles that can bring some clarification to these hard issues of policy? The following are starters. They will not automatically resolve policy problems. But they—and undoubtedly other principles which should be added—might help to bring some needed perspectives to the policy dilemmas.

1. Do not separate individual rights and social good from each other. In the vision of the good community, a foretaste of the Commonwealth of God, there can be no such division. A utilitarian cost-benefit analysis, so frequently employed in policy decisions, always risks the violation of this principle. At best such utilitarian calculus will maximize the fundamental issues of society at large. It seldom offers protection for the rights of minorities. Thus, to those who propose that we quarantine all persons with AIDS, let the question be asked: In addition to the fundamental violation of civil liberties this would involve, what would such a policy do to the whole fabric of society? In addition to the enormous personal costs to those affected, what would be the social costs if resources were spent on quarantine? What might be the costs to everyone's liberty? Do we want to live in such a society?

Note that questions such as these involve both individual rights and social good. That is utterly appropriate, and the bias is in the direction of a "no quarantine" judgment. But now, what if the question is not that of quarantining *all* persons with AIDS, but rather just *one*? The man who insists upon continuing his work of male prostitution after a positive diagnosis? The case is not fictional. The decision is difficult. The lesson, I believe, is that no rule is absolute, even a no-quarantine rule. But, however the difficult cases are decided, neither the social good nor individual rights ought to be considered or emphasized apart from each other.

2. Consciously test each policy proposal for elements of homophobia, and racism as well. Because of these elements, this epidemic is different from any other we have faced. For example, a false-but-powerful contagion theory has long operated concerning sexual orientation ("If we allow gay and lesbian teachers into our elementary schools, our children will 'catch it' "). Now, in spite of clear medical information to the contrary, such contagion fears unconsciously and strongly lap over into AIDS issues ("Don't let that child with AIDS into my child's school"). The insidious and distorting power of homophobic fears needs constant reminder and vigilance.

3. Presume in favor of oppressed minorities. "God's preferential option for the oppressed" is one of liberation theology's important recoveries from the prophetic biblical tradition. Such a perspective leads to a certain burden-of-proof mentality in assessing policies. There is a presumption in favor of those who are most likely to be hurt. They have already been discriminated against by social structures and practices. Thus, in formulating policies relating to AIDS for cities, state health departments, hospitals, and community agencies, it is extraordinarily important that members of AIDS high-risk groups be strongly represented and carefully heard in all deliberations.

4. Ensure as much self-control as possible by those most directly affected in the execution of policies. The policy of "contact notification" is a case in point. Gay and bisexual men realistically fear possession by the State of sexual contact names. On the other hand, public health officials (also with some realism) fear that if sexual contact notification is left entirely to the individual's own motivation and sense of responsibility, in some cases it will not happen. But a public agency might contract with a private organization (gay-controlled and gay-trusted) to undertake followup tracing and notifying of sexual contacts. Granted, legal problems would have to be ironed out in this arrangement, but they are not insuperable. The benefits are worth it. The trust and cooperation of the gay community is absolutely essential if this and other measures are to work.

5. Avoid moralizing the issue at hand. "Moralizing" means the tendency to sacrifice larger issues of justice and well-being in favor of controlling certain behaviors of which one does not approve. Some people are offended by frank "safer sex" education. But only that educational approach which is sufficiently explicit and erotically appealing may be effective. Yes, some people are offended by the image of sex in the bathhouse. But, as argued above, closing bathhouses may actually be counterproductive in modifying high-risk sexual behaviors, in addition to being a questionable violation of personal rights. Or—to shift the focus to another, if small, high-risk group—some may be offended by the public provision of free sanitary needles to I.V. drug users. But the withholding of needles will scarcely modify the drug practice. Their provision might significantly slow this source of

AIDS transmission.

The Church's Creative Repentance

We who call ourselves Christian bear major responsibility
for the problems created by the AIDS crisis. Over the centuries we have given considerable religious sanction to
homophobia. We have been the major institutional
legitimizer of compulsory heterosexuality—and the punisher
of those who did not conform to that heterosexual norm. Our
metanoia, our creative repentance, calls us to constructive
responses to the current tragedy.

To date, with the notable exceptions of some gay-lesbian
ministries—the Universal Fellowship of Metropolitan Community Churches, and a few scattered urban mainline churches—the response of most church bodies has been hesi-
tant and tardy. Some of the needs are clear: Like any other
problem of human suffering and social complexity, the AIDS
situation calls for acts of compassion, sensitivity, level-
headedness, and informed public advocacy. A good place to
begin is education and communication about the disease
and the needs of those most affected, especially in cooperation with members of the high risk groups themselves. Further, direct acts of caring, service, and compassion are obviously needed, in volunteers for home care, hospitals,
hospices, and for support for other care-givers.

Sensitive pastoral care and counseling for those directly
affected by the disease are urgent needs. These pastoral
needs extend to the families of persons with AIDS. For
some, the diagnosis of the disease will also reveal for the
first time a son's, brother's, or husband's sexual orientation.
If public policies and agencies are to be mobilized more fully, enormous tasks of advocacy need to be undertaken.

POLITICS OF AIDS

AN INFORMED SOCIETY'S RESPONSE: THE POINT

William E. Dannemeyer

William E. Dannemeyer is a conservative republican representative from the thirty-ninth congressional district in California. The following comments were made at a symposium on AIDS at Stanford University.

Points to Consider

1. How have public health authorities responded to the AIDS disease?
2. What is the ELISA test and how effective is it?
3. Why should bathhouses be closed down?
4. How should health care workers with AIDS be dealt with?
5. Why should children with AIDS not be allowed to attend school?

Excerpted from a speech by William E. Dannemeyer, Stanford University Symposium on AIDS, January 24, 1986.

AIDS is a virus and viruses do not have civil rights.

We have learned much about AIDS. We know that it is incurable, contagious and 100% fatal. We know that it is typically transmitted through sexual contact, intravenous drug use and exposure to infected blood. We also know that there are more than 17,000 confirmed cases of AIDS in the United States and that there may be as many as 2 million carriers. Although we have come a long way, there is still much we don't know.

What we do know is that inaction is not a substitute for cure. As a society we must pursue measures to protect the public health of the nation while continuing our research efforts to find a vaccine and a cure.

The failure of our public health authorities to take anything more than "symbolic" steps in confronting this crisis can be at least partially attributed to efforts by civil rights activists to characterize any efforts to protect the public health as an attempt to infringe upon the civil rights of AIDS victims. AIDS is a virus and viruses do not have civil rights. With an epidemic of these proportions, we are faced with a real threat to our society and must err, if we are to err at all, on the side of caution, not play Russian roulette with the unknown.

While we await a cure for this deadly disease, we are faced with difficult issues and public policy choices. As a Member of Congress, I have introduced five bills to ensure that the public's health is not compromised by inaction. These measures address crucial questions involving the integrity of our blood supply, bathhouses, the health care industry and school-age victims of AIDS.

I. Safety of the Blood Supply

The percentage of AIDS cases related to contaminated blood has doubled since 1984 from 1% to 2% (261 adults and 33 children). Although transfusion recipients represent the smallest high-risk groups for AIDS, the existence of this group brings into question the integrity of our blood supply and the credibility of CDC authorities who avow the "complete safety" and reliability of the nation's blood banks.

120

The ELISA test, now used by all blood banks as a screening device, represents an important step in screening out contaminated blood. It is not foolproof however, and has been shown to produce a false negative result in 3-4% of screenings for contaminated blood. Recently, a number of prominent scientists have been questioning its reliability. Among them is Dr. Alvin Novak, an AIDS researcher at Yale University, who said that the claims of reliability from the Centers for Disease Control (CDC) are "grossly inaccurate and at best misleading" and that the ELISA test could fail up to 10% of the time.

CDC initially issued guidelines for blood donation on February 14, 1985, prohibiting intravenous drug users and Haitians from donating blood and requesting male homosexuals who had not been monogamous since 1979 to refrain from donating. These guidelines were issued despite the fact that a Kinsey Study showed that the average relationship between male homosexuals was 1 to 3 years and that they were generally not monogamous. In August, I wrote to Margaret Heckler, then Secretary of Health and Human Services, to request that these guidelines be changed to *prohibit* all male homosexuals from donating blood. On September 6, CDC's guidelines were changed to partially accommodate my recommendation and *request* that any male who has had sex with another male since 1977 *refrain* from donating blood. In October, some chapters of the American Red Cross implemented some changes of their own and affixed a sticker to the front of their blood donation literature which reads: "males who have had sex with another male since 1977 *must not* donate blood". Just since the first of the year, they have started distributing a new brochure nationally which finally states that males who have had sex with other males since 1977 must not donate blood. While I am encouraged by these actions, I feel several steps are still in order.

First, I feel that since male homosexuals comprise the largest high-risk AIDS group (73%), they should be prohibited from donating and must be placed in the same category as intravenous drug users.

Secondly, since the integrity of the blood supply is still at issue, I believe facilities should be made available to individuals wishing to pursue autologous and directed blood donations. When an individual knows he may need a transfusion, as in the case of elective surgery, he should have the option of earmarking his own blood, or the blood of a relative for his specific use should the need arise.

Lastly, I have introduced legislation, H.R. 3649, which makes it a crime for those who know that they are members of an AIDS high-risk group to donate blood. The purpose of this legislation is to give some "teeth" to CDC guidelines and provide a legal deterrent to individuals tempted to practice "blood terrorism". This bill has been referred to the Judiciary Committee and hearings have been requested.

II. Close Down Bathhouses

Another issue which public health authorities have sidestepped in their efforts to avoid a civil rights confrontation is the closure of homosexual bathhouses. We know that male homosexuals comprise 73% of all AIDS cases, that in many large cities the majority of male homosexuals have been exposed to the virus, that AIDS is transmitted through sexual contact and that anonymous sexual contact with a number of partners occurs routinely in bathhouses. Despite the impeccable logic behind closing these establishments, public health authorities have failed to recommend or implement this action.

In August of 1985, Congress overwhelmingly voted to give the Surgeon General the power to close bathhouses. Despite this almost unanimous show of support, no additional action has been taken. For that reason I introduced H.R. 3648 which would cut off federal revenue sharing funds to cities which fail to close public bathhouses deemed to be a health hazard.

III. Health Care Industry

The health care industry is of particular concern due to the vulnerability of patients during a time of illness. We know that AIDS is transmitted through the exchange of body fluids. We also know that health care providers are in intimate contact with the blood, secretions, tears and saliva of patients on a regular basis.

The duties of health care workers place them in direct contact with vulnerable individuals more likely to contract opportunistic infections than the general population. Health care workers daily perform a variety of at-risk activities including inserting IV's, coming into contact with secretions, performing mouth-to-mouth resuscitation and performing other intimate services which place at risk the health of the patient as well as the health of the worker/victim. Based on my meeting with nurses from San Francisco General Hospital and testimony from nurses before the Republican Study Committee of the House, I introduced two bills to deal with the problem of AIDS in the health care industry.

H.R. 3647 prohibits health care workers with AIDS from working in the health care delivery system and cuts off federal funds to those hospitals which fail to do so. This action seems only prudent when victims of AIDS carry a number of attendant diseases which are themselves contagious, including such diseases as amebiosis, giardiasis (gay bowel syndrome) and cytomegalovirus, all of which may be socially transmitted. . . .

These persons should not be placed in responsible jobs where the lives and health of other individuals are at stake.

In addition, by its nature a virus is capable of mutation which means that at some point what we now know about routes of transmission may no longer hold true. An article in the September 28, 1985 issue of the respected British medical journal *The Lancet,* reported that, contrary to U.S. medical reports, the AIDS virus can live up to 10 days at room temperature outside the body and still remain virulent. This study brings into question whether the exchange of

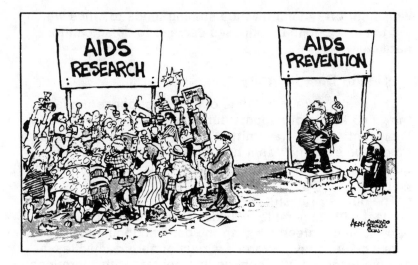

body fluids is the only method of transmission or merely the most likely. In light of this study and the disagreement in the medical community about the virulence of AIDS, we must exercise caution and take steps to protect those most unable to protect themselves.

I have also introduced H.R. 3646 which authorizes health care professionals to use their discretion in wearing protective garments when treating AIDS patients. This proposal is a result of my meetings with nurses from San Francisco General Hospital who were prohibited by superiors from wearing protective garments when dealing with AIDS patients because this practice reportedly "impinged on the sensitivities of the AIDS patient". Nurses are trained in the management of infectious disease and should be allowed to exercise their professional judgement in protecting themselves and their patients from the threat of contracting AIDS or any other infectious illness. When faced with a choice, the protection of our health care professionals must be a priority.

IV. School Children

We know that at least 231 children are the unfortunate victims of AIDS. What we don't know is how many more children will be faced with this deadly disease before we

124

have a cure or how effectively children with AIDS will be able to protect themselves and their classmates in a situation which places both parties at risk.

To its credit, CDC addressed this subject and issued guidelines for schools to follow should a school-age child be diagnosed with AIDS. To its discredit, CDC's guidelines failed to provide any rational recommendations to aid school officials in making a determination. CDC's guidelines suggest that a child with AIDS should remain in the classroom absent exceptional circumstances or illustrations of unusual, high-risk behavior such as biting, scratching or vomitting. Essentially, these guidelines suggest that a child's propensity for biting, scratching or vomitting should be apparent upon consultation with the child.

I reject that approach. Such a policy places the life of the AIDS child at risk and places the lives of the other children in a position of potential peril. We don't know that the disease can be transmitted by these behaviors and we don't know that it can't. Until concerned parents can be guaranteed that there is no risk to their child in attending school with a child with AIDS, I believe we must adopt a cautious approach to protect all concerned. To date, no medical authorities have issued this guarantee. For that reason I introduced H. Con. Res. 224 which expresses the sense of Congress that children with AIDS should not attend school and should be provided alternative forms of education.

V. Quarantine

It has frequently been reported that I support the use of quarantine to control the spread of the AIDS virus. Those reports are unfounded. *I do not and never have called for or endorsed the idea of quarantine of AIDS victims or any others to control this epidemic.* To have any chance of being effective, quarantine would require taking away the civil rights of as many as a million Americans for an extended period of time, perhaps for life, be extremely expensive, and of questionable benefit. Therefore, a combination of the actions which I have recommended above and effective, consistent, and on going education of all Americans, especially those at high risk, are the only realistic approaches now available to combat the spread of AIDS.

One other step is necessary. We must find a way to change the approach of this nation's public health officials. They have not treated AIDS like other epidemics or even like other venereal diseases. AIDS has been accorded special prominence as a public health issue—which is appropriate— and special privileges as a civil rights issue—which is not. AIDS is a public health crisis of epidemic proportions, not a civil rights battle.

Public health officials attempting to control the spread of a contagious venereal disease routinely contact the sexual partners of infected individuals and even isolate infected individuals who fail to refrain from prohibited sexual activities. Although the same powers are in place for controlling the spread of AIDS, they have not been exercised, apparently because of the prevailing fear that such acts will be deemed civil rights violations.

The role of public health authorities is to contain this disease. AIDS should be accorded the same stature as other epidemics and public health authorities should not bow to powerful public pressure and coercive lobbying efforts to alter the course of appropriate and necessary public policy in the name of civil rights.

Although there are those who have questioned the motives of a politician and candidate for the United States Senate speaking out on a public health issue and calling medical professionals and public health officers to task for their lack of action, I assure you that I have not attempted to use AIDS as a political issue. There is too great a risk of bringing suffering, fear and pain to too many people for this to be allowed to become a partisan issue. However, it is also too important an issue to all of us for me to be willing to avoid discussing it and calling for necessary action just to avoid accusations.

We cannot afford the luxury of ignoring AIDS and hoping that it will go away. As a public official, I cannot allow myself the luxury of being silent. If we do not take definitive action NOW, even actions which will compromise some of the rights of some in our society, we risk the very real possibility of disaster in this country. Let us not take this threat too lightly.

POLITICS OF AIDS

AN INFORMED SOCIETY'S RESPONSE: THE COUNTERPOINT

National Gay & Lesbian Task Force

The National Gay & Lesbian Task Force has been active in the area of funding and supporting civil rights issues concerning AIDS since 1981.

Points to Consider

1. What is the HTLV-III antibody test?
2. What dangers does this test present?
3. How are the Public Health Service Occupational Guidelines for Prevention of AIDS described?
4. Why are gay organizations opposed to government regulations of sexual behavior in bathhouses and related establishments?

Excerpted from position papers by the National Gay & Lesbian Task Force, 1985, 1986.

There is no medical basis for denying employment to people with AIDS, ARC, or HTLV-III infection as long as they are well enough to perform their duties.

As soon as AIDS became established as an epidemic in this country, organizations concerned with the civil rights of Americans began to receive reports of discrimination—in employment, insurance, housing, health care, and government services—against persons with AIDS and members of the groups at increased risk. This new problem emerges in the context of a long standing pattern of discrimination against lesbians and gay men on the basis of their sexual orientation; the discrimination is sometimes subtle, sometimes overt, other times brutal, involving physical violence. That 73% of the AIDS cases in the U.S. have been observed among bisexual and homosexual males has provided the bigoted with a new excuse for discrimination against the members of our community. NGTF, through its Crisisline, has been taking reports of AIDS-related discrimination and providing the victims with referrals.

The test for antibodies to HTLV-III, just entering widespread use, increases the potential for AIDS-related discrimination. There is wide-spread concern in the gay and lesbian community that public hysteria might influence public policy in the direction of unjustifiable actions against persons with AIDS or persons testing positive on the antibody test as a class. Consequently, efforts to maintain lists of persons identified as being antibody positive, however benevolent the intentions behind such actions and however good the confidentiality safeguards, are viewed with much trepidation. . . .

The HTLV-III Antibody Test

As a result of negotiations between the Food and Drug Administration and NGTF and Lambda Legal Defense and Education Fund, there is labeling associated with the test that can be used as a tool to prevent or take action against misuse.

128

The labeling states that the test does not diagnose AIDS and should not be used as a general screen for AIDS or to identify individuals in high risk groups. In other words, this test should not be used to promote discrimination against gay men and others at risk to AIDS. (There is of course a limited and valid use of this test to screen blood and blood products). *We urge you to monitor use of this test in your community* and identify those clinics, laboratories, and physicians who misrepresent the usefulness of the test. For example, anyone who advertises the availability of the antibody test using terms like "AIDS screening" or "AIDS testing" is violating the labeling associated with the test. You should attempt to correct this misrepresentation at the local level, but we also urge you to inform the Food and Drug Administration of this misuse, since they have the capability of taking steps against those who violate the labeling restrictions.

We also urge you to take several preventative steps against misuse. These include obtaining advisory rulings from human rights/civil rights and insurance regulatory agencies warning employers and insurance companies that this test should not become part of any of their screening procedures. Your jurisdiction need not have gay/lesbian civil rights protections in order for use of this test to be considered a violation of the rights of an employee or an applicant for insurance. . . .

Blood Testing in the Military

Regrettably, the Defense Department has announced that all prospective recruits will be screened for antibody to HTLV-III. The military did not bother to wait for the recommendation of the Armed Services Epidemiological Board (before which NGTF [National Gay Task Force] had testified—see release dated Aug. 13). Though the circumstances of employment within the military are special— live virus vaccines that might possibly harm the immune-deficient are routinely administered to new recruits and battlefield situations sometimes require emergency transfusions from one soldier to another—the Pentagon's action may encourage the use of the test in civilian employment screening. The Pentagon's medical department has indicated that it will reconsider an applicant if additional testing in-

New Medicines

Despite the public uproar over AIDS, we have not yet focused on the key questions: How do we discover new medicines to help sick people, and what can we do to encourage and speed up such discoveries against AIDS and other killing or crippling ailments?

Harry Schwartz, New York Times, *September 6, 1985*

dicates that their immune system is not seriously impaired, though given their long-standing discriminatory stance, there is reason to be skeptical of this claim. Those contemplating joining the armed services and anxious about their antibody status should be advised that they can get the test in advance at an Alternative Testing Site where it is available with confidentiality protections. As of the moment, current military personnel are not going to be screened, but this situation could change. . . .

Occupational Guidelines for Prevention of AIDS

On November 18, 1985, the Public Health Service published recommendations covering the risk of transmitting the virus associated with AIDS, HTLV-III/LAV, in the workplace. (The text was published in the CDC's *Morbidity and Mortality Report*). These landmark guidelines cover all occupations except surgeons and dentists engaged in "invasive" procedures (which are in preparation). They are unequivocal in stating that, apart from the very small and avoidable risk faced by health-care workers in terms of needlestick injuries, there is *no* risk of transmitting AIDS in the workplace—from employee to client or vice versa—and therefore no medical basis for denying employment or services to people with AIDS, or HTLV-III/LAV infection.

This is a sound scientific document based on all available epidemiologic and other medical data. There is still no evidence to suggest that HTLV-III/LAV is transmitted other than through the three known routes: sexual intercourse, injection with blood or blood components (a route largely limited to IV drug use, now that effective screening procedures are in use for the blood supply), and from mother to fetus/newborn infant. As noted in the guidelines and as already published elsewhere, "studies of non-sexual household contacts of AIDS patients indicate that casual contact with saliva and tears does not result in transmission or infection."

Of particular interest to the communities most affected by AIDS:

• The guidelines "do *not* recommend routine HTLV-III/LAV antibody screening for the groups addressed [which include health-care, food-service, and personal-service workers] . . . because AIDS is not spread by casual contact."

• There is no medical basis for denying employment to people with AIDS, ARC, or HTLV-III infection as long as they are well enough to perform their duties, since "the kind of non-sexual person to person contact that generally occurs among workers and clients or consumers in the workplace does not pose a risk for transmission of HTLV-III/LAV."

• There is no basis for concern about transmission from worker to client and client to worker as long as standard precautions for each occupation are taken. No extraordinary measures are necessary for health-care workers, personal-service workers (hairdressers, manicurists, masseurs, etc.), or food-service workers.

• Of 1,498 health care workers accidentally exposed to body fluids of patients with AIDS, only two—both needlestick injuries—appear to have developed antibodies to HTLV-III/LAV as a result and neither of these have developed AIDS.

• There is no evidence of transmission having occurred in even a single instance from health-care worker (HCW) to patient, from personal-service worker (PSW) to client, or from food-service worker (FSW) to consumer.

• The guidelines emphasize that "because the hepatitis B virus is also bloodborne and both hardier and more infectious than HTLV-III/LAV, recommendations that would prevent the transmission of hepatitis B will also prevent transmission of AIDS" in health-care and certain personal-service (acupuncture, tattooing, ear-piercing, etc.) settings.

• Appropriate precautions based on the hepatitis B model are once again outlined for health-care workers in institutional, home care, and pre-hospital emergency settings. . . .

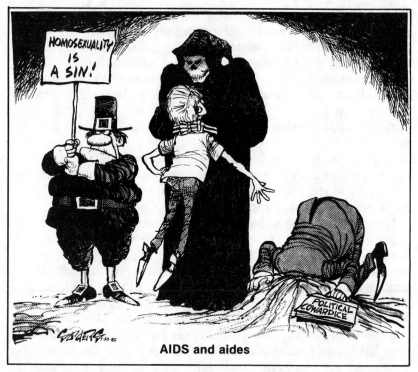

AIDS and aides

By Bill Sanders, *Milwaukee Journal.* Permission of News America Syndicate.

These guidelines should become an invaluable tool in fighting discrimination in the workplace. They should be used as an authoritative, independent, public health assessment for fighting restrictions on the employment of persons with AIDS or ARC or positive antibody test results who are able to work. They provide the arguments needed against such measures as mandatory testing (involving "health cards" or other identifying records) that might be suggested as requirements for food service, personal service, or health care workers. . . .

Government Regulations

The National Gay Task Force stands opposed to government regulations that attempt to police the sexual behavior of individuals in bathhouses and related establishments and objects to the closure of any establishment based on the violation of such regulations. We are concerned that the regulatory actions taken in San Francisco and New York establish a dangerous precedent in favor of the reinstitution of sodomy statues and other violations of the right to privacy. We fear that these regulations might be extended to infringe on the right of freedom of association in those places (e.g., churches, coffeehouses, and most bars) where sexual activity does not take place but where gay men and lesbians seek refuge from a hostile society. Government can play a constructive role in preventing AIDS: by funding expanded educational programs to promote safe sexual activity. The regulatory powers of government may legitimately extend to enforcing educational, structural, and hygienic standards in the operation of bathhouses and related establishments, but should not extend to the direct or indirect coercion of individuals.

Across the country, local and state governments are, in response to increased public concern—sometimes escalating to hysteria—considering what actions they might take to diminish the spread of the virus associated with AIDS, including the regulation or closure of establishments, such as bathhouses, that have traditionally catered to sexual activity that now presents a significant risk of transmitting AIDS.

Constructive Role

There *is* a constructive role government can play in promoting the prevention of AIDS in the context of such establishments. It can support, through funding for prevention education, expanded efforts in such establishments to persuade the ever-diminishing minority within the gay male community which continues to engage in high-risk sexual activity to follow safe sex guidelines. Government can also legitimately regulate these businesses as it regulates other businesses; this could extend to precise operating standards involving educational, structural, and hygienic requirements, but should not extend to government policing of individual behavior on the premises. Government can legitimately close a publicly licensed establishment if (after it has been given the opportunity to comply) it does not adhere to reasonable regulations including, e.g., adequate lighting, hygiene, and rigorous on-site education to promote safe sexual activity. Government need not and should not be taking actions that amount to the direct policing of private adult consensual behavior. . . .

As an organization concerned not only with public health and the fight against AIDS but also with civil liberties, we are concerned that the logic employed in regulations could be extended to justify reinstitution of "sodomy statutes" (proscribing behavior under any circumstances—even in the privacy of one's home) in those 25 states where homosexual conduct is not currently illegal, or the active enforcement of such statutes where they still exist. There are already indications that New York state is considering the monitoring of hotel rooms where certain sexual acts may be occurring behind closed doors, a course of action that could carry regulations well beyond the regulation of sex clubs and bathhouses and which could ultimately threaten the right to privacy of all citizens, gay and straight. . . .

These regulations might furthermore be used as a precedent to justify the closure or regulatory harrassment of establishments where sexual activity does *not* take place—e.g. Metropolitan Community Churches (MCC), coffeehouses, offices of student gay organizations, and most bars—but where gay men go to seek refuge from a society that is often hostile and unaccepting. In some parts of the country, the right to freedom of association of gay men and lesbians for the purposes of social support is regularly violated, a situation that prevailed prior to the epidemic but is now sometimes "justified" by concerns over AIDS. . . .

It is important for government agencies to recognize that education, though grossly underfunded, has been successful in helping to bring about the significant changes that have taken place among gay men collectively since the AIDS epidemic was recognized in early 1982. . . .

A recent study revealed that among a broad-based sample of gay men 81% are currently not engaging in sexual activity that might place themselves or others at risk for exposure to the virus associated with AIDS. . . .

Conclusion

State and local governments should also recognize that forced closure, as opposed to reasonable efforts to regulate these establishments, may yield short-term political advantages, but will not in itself result in the elimination of the transmission of HTLV-III, even within the gay male community, and may in fact foster the development of an underground of establishments that would be relatively immune to any kind of regulation and community-based educational efforts.

Any contemplated regulations should apply and be enforced equally with respect to establishments that cater to sexually active heterosexuals. They should be prepared in consultation with the AIDS service organizations that now exist in virtually every city with a significant incidence of this disease.

It is our belief that through concerted and innovative educational programs AIDS service organizations and the public health agencies with which they cooperate, can help an every-increasing proportion of sexually active gay men to understand and follow safe sex guidelines. Such programs must also reach out to gay youth and all those others who are just now coming out as gay men and who face critical choices that will effect their future well-being.

It is our hope that the controversy revolving around the fate of establishments permitting sexual activity to take place on their premises will not obscure the very real and serious affronts to civil rights—discrimination in employment and insurance—that currently menace every person at increased risk for AIDS, and which demand protective measures from government.

POLITICS OF AIDS

PROHIBITING DISCRIMINATION

Charles Cooper

Is AIDS considered a handicap under federal law? Responding to a request for legal advice from Ronald Robertson, general counsel for the Department of Health and Human Services, Assistant Attorney General Charles Cooper signed a 49-page opinion which interprets legal rights of people with AIDS. The opinion interprets those rights much more narrowly than the Justice Department's career civil rights lawyers had recommended.

Protection to AIDS victims is provided by federal civil rights laws. However, the Justice Department's ruling permits employers and public health officials who believe they are preventing the spread of AIDS, to dismiss a person with acquired immune deficiency syndrome.

According to the opinion, if an AIDS victim is excluded from a federal program or dismissed from a job solely because he suffers from the disease, the exclusion or dismissal would be illegal. If he were excluded or dismissed because of concern that the victim might spread the disease to others then the exclusion or dismissal would not necessarily be illegal.

The Justice Department pointed out the importance of making the distinction between recognizing the disabling effects of the disease on its victim and the ability to spread the condition to others. The opinion is binding on the executive branch of government.

Charles Cooper, Department of Justice Opinion, June 20, 1986.

Points to Consider

1. Under what circumstances is it illegal to fire a person with AIDS?
2. Under what circumstances is it legal to fire a person with AIDS?
3. What is the Rehabilitation Act of 1973?
4. How old are laws to prevent the spread of contagious diseases?

We have concluded that an individual's (real or perceived) ability to transmit the disease to others is not a handicap.

In a letter of March 11, 1986, you asked this Office to consider a variety of questions concerning the application of section 504 of the Rehabilitation Act of 1973, to individuals who have (or are regarded as having) Acquired Immune Deficiency Syndrome ("AIDS") or AIDS-related complex ("ARC") or who test positive for AIDS antibodies. Section 504 prohibits discrimination based solely on handicap against any otherwise qualified person in any program that is conducted by the federal government or that receives federal assistance. You have informed us that your Department's Office of Civil Rights has received complaints in which workers employed in hospitals or clinics allege that they have been discriminated against by their employers because they fall within or are regarded as falling within these categories.

Major Findings

After carefully examining these difficult questions, we have concluded that section 504 prohibits discrimination based on the disabling effects that AIDS and related conditions may have on their victims. By contrast, we have concluded that an individual's (real or perceived) ability to transmit the disease to others is not a handicap within the meaning of the statute and, therefore, that discrimination on this basis does not fall within section 504. This conclusion is compelled not only by the statute's language, but also by sound and frequently invoked principles of statutory interpretation. In particular, we find it highly significant that Congress, in enacting section 504, gave no indication that it intended to disturb the venerable body of federal and state law giving public health officials broad powers to prevent the spread of communicable diseases. We accordingly are convinced that no such change was intended.

This opinion is limited to an examination of section 504, which serves the highly important, but limited, role of prohibiting discrimination based on handicap in covered programs and activities. We have not examined any other federal, state, or local laws that may extend broader protections in this field. . . .

Pretext for Discrimination

It should be noted that the reasonableness of an employer's concern about the spread of disease is relevant only to the extent it bears on the question of pretext. As we have shown, section 504 simply does not reach decisions based on fear of contagion—whether reasonable or not—so long as it is not in truth a pretext for discrimination on account of handicap. An employer, for example, who makes hiring decisions based on an unreasonable concern about contagion is no different from an employer whose hiring decisions rest on any other unreasonable basis that lies outside section 504's limited reach. To illustrate this point, consider an employer who has the bizarre belief that persons with curly hair make better employees than persons with straight hair. . . . Section 504 does not prohibit the employer from making hiring decisions based on this wholly unreasonable basis. Straight hair is not a handicap; nor is

138

discrimination against such persons conceivably a pretext masking discrimination against the handicapped. Therefore, discrimination against persons with straight hair, as irrational and deplorable as it may be, is not within section 504's scope.

Consequently, there is no a priori reason to presume that assertions of fear of contagion of AIDS are especially likely to be pretextual. Whatever the medical facts regarding transmissibility might be, a constellation of factors make it intuitively plausible that a person claiming fear of contagion genuinely discriminated on that basis rather than by reason of handicap. The consequences of contracting the virus are severe; there is a substantial chance, possibly even approaching 100%, that the infected individual will eventually contract the disease. And the disease itself is both incurable and fatal—it appears that everyone who contracts it will die. In common experience, even a very low probability of contracting a contagious virus with consequences of this magnitude is likely to call forth a strongly-felt response. In addition, there are a number of questions regarding AIDS on which the medical community does not speak with one voice. Knowledge of the disease is growing and, in some respects, changing rapidly. The mechanisms of transmission are still not fully understood, and epidemiological evidence does not permit the kind of categorical statements about risk that would make one doubt the legitimacy of claims of fear. These considerations must inform any analysis engaged in by a factfinder to determine whether discrimination truly occurred by reason of handicap, and thus counsel against an initial presumption of pretext. . . .

Extent of Harm

Obviously, the extent of the harm that would be caused by a contagious disease bears an inverse relationship to the degree of risk of transmission that a normal person would be willing, or can be required, to assume. For example, the common cold is highly contagious, and the mechanism of its transmission is well known and commonly understood. Its consequences, however, are typically temporary and not severe, and most people will not go to extraordinary lengths to avoid exposure to a significant risk of infection. At the other end of the spectrum would be a contagious disease that is incurable, highly painful, and ultimately fatal. The typical human response to such a disease is to take substantial measures to avoid exposure to even the slightest risk of infection. This natural tendency to "err on the safe side" when dealing with such a disease is compounded when, as with AIDS, the state of medical knowledge concerning it is still in an early stage of development, and the mechanisms of the disease's transmission are not fully understood.

We do not believe that Congress intended enactment of section 504 substantially to rearrange human conduct with regard to contagious illnesses. . . .

Our conclusion that section 504 does not reach discrimination based on communicability finds emphatic support in the statute's legislative history, particularly when viewed against the background of existing laws dealing with this subject.

Because of the enormous damage wrought by epidemics of contagious diseases, "measures to prevent the spread of dangerous communicable diseases. . . .are practically as old as history.". . . For centuries, Anglo-American law has given

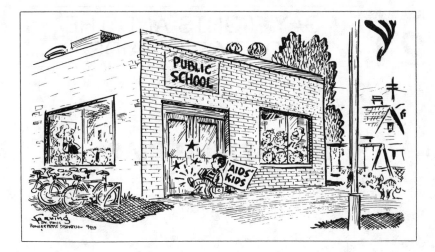

public health officials broad authority to deal with communicable diseases through quarantine and other measures. The very first crime discussed by William Blackstone in the chapter of his *Commentaries on the Law of England* dealing with offenses against the public health, police, or economy is disobedience of a quarantine order. . . .

Conclusion

For the foregoing reasons, we conclude that discrimination based on the disabling effects of AIDS on its victims may violate section 504, but that the statute does not restrict measures taken to prevent the spread of the disease. This Memorandum, of course, does not purport to answer all questions concerning the relationship between section 504 and AIDS, but we trust that our analysis will be helpful to you in resolving the difficult questions that you face.

GAY RIGHTS AND THE POLITICS OF AIDS

UNLEASHING BIAS

The Nation

The following statement was excerpted from an article by the editors of The Nation, *a liberal magazine of social and political opinion.*

Points to Consider

1. How is the Justice Department ruling on the rights of AIDS patients defined?
2. How has this ruling legitimized AIDS hysteria?
3. What are the other implications of the Justice Department ruling?
4. What has happened to AIDS patients in nursing homes and hospitals?

In a single ruling, and against every shred of reliable medical opinion, the Justice Department has legitimized AIDS hysteria.

The Justice Department's ruling on the rights of AIDS patients doubles their distress by putting them at risk of discrimination at the same time that they are victims of disease. Assistant Attorney General for Civil Rights William Bradford Reynolds apparently overrode the objections of virtually every career lawyer and many recent appointees in his division to place the government on record against classifying AIDS as a handicap, which would have triggered the application of non-discrimination guarantees under Federal law. Even those who are not sick but who test positive for HTLV-III virus are denied their civil rights. In a single ruling, and against every shred of reliable medical opinion, the Justice Department has legitimized AIDS hysteria and has given employers, landlords, school administrators and social-service bureaucrats the right to create a pariah class of Americans.

In March the Department of Health and Human Services asked Justice whether AIDS patients met the 1973 Rehabilitation Act's definition of a handicapped person, that is, one whose physical impairment substantially limits one or more "major life activities." Until now it was believed that serious chronic infectious diseases, such as tuberculosis and virally induced cancers, were covered by the statute. No one argued that protection against discrimination allowed sick people to communicate their disease to others. If there is no significant danger of infection, however, those handicapped by illness should not be denied protection under the law.

Casual Contact

The Centers for Disease Control and the Public Health Service, as well as private physicians in every major locality affected by AIDS, agree that the syndrome cannot be transmitted by casual contact and that it is, in fact, less communicable than many viral and sexually transmitted

143

diseases. Some courts have ruled that children with AIDS, a growing category of victims, cannot be barred from school. But the Justice Department says that the fear of catching the disease is enough to sanction discrimination unless that fear is merely "a pretext for discrimination on account of handicap." Furthermore, a positive antibody test result may be a legitimate ground for discrimination. The person with AIDS, or the one who is seropositive for the virus, must prove that he or she is not contagious and that the discriminatory act was motivated purely by prejudice due to the disability. Patients would then have to pursue their rights through the Reagan court system, not an optimistic prospect.

While certain sympathetic officials in Health and Human Services and other government bureaus try to get Reynolds to soften his stand, the impact of the ruling is being discussed and analyzed throughout the medical and the civil liberties community. First off, it's clear that the government's position has implications that go beyond AIDS. In the past few years, and often as a result of AIDS research, scientists have lengthened the list of diseases known to be caused, or in some way induced, by infectious agents. Ulcers, some

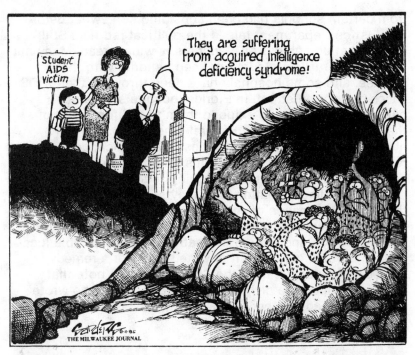

By Bill Sanders, *Milwaukee Journal.* Permission of News America Syndicate.

leukemias, many other cancers and perhaps multiple sclerosis and auto-immune disorders seem to be linked to infection. Within a few years, it may be possible to detect genetic markers in otherwise healthy individuals for a range of illnesses that will produce handicaps and serious functional impairments later in their lives. Logically, anyone with an infectious disease or with a marker for a disease may be subject to sanctioned discrimination, at least under the Justice Department's AIDS guidelines. Legal and medical counselors are already advising clients in high-risk categories to refrain from taking the AIDS virus test, which offers no help in treatment and which may well be used to discriminate against them in work, residence, education or health care.

Hysteria

The hysteria that infected the country last summer after Rock Hudson's death and the exclusion of pupils with AIDS from certain schools had been subsiding somewhat before the Justice Department raised the political red flag. Still, discrimination against AIDS victims is widespread. Many nursing homes refuse to admit or keep patients with the disease, and some hospitals have been throwing their AIDS cases out on the street. In Florida, hospitals have put patients on planes and shipped them to California. All of these institutions receive Federal funds, and all are prohibited from discriminating against the handicapped. As a result of the Justice Department's ruling, those with AIDS will be severely restricted in seeking redress.

Local antidiscrimination laws may still apply to AIDS patients, but thousands of very sick people are likely to get caught in the crossfire between a prejudiced and vindictive Administration and a more sympathetic but vulnerable local service bureaucracy. And if anyone hopes for a remedy, someday, somehow, from the Supreme Court, note that Charles Cooper, the civil rights division lawyer who wrote the ruling, used to clerk for the designated Chief Justice of the United States.

GAY RIGHTS AND THE
POLITICS OF AIDS

POINTS AND COUNTERPOINTS: SHOULD SODOMY BE PROTECTED BY THE CONSTITUTION?

Justice White vs Justice Stevens

The Supreme Court ruled on June 30, 1986 that there is no constitutionally protected right to engage in homosexual conduct between consenting adults, even in their homes. The court upheld a Georgia law that makes it a criminal act for men or women to engage in anal or oral sex. The majority said the ruling involved only the rights of a homosexual man in Atlanta. It did not rule on whether married and heterosexual couples were constitutionally protected from prosecution under this same Georgia law.

The case ruled on by the Court was a civil suit challenging Georgia's sodomy law. This suit was brought by Michael Harding. He is a homosexual, arrested in his Atlanta bedroom while having sexual relations with another man. A police officer had come to Hardwick's house to serve a warrant because he had not paid a fine for public drunkenness. The person who answered the door gave the police officer permission to find Hardwick. Although he was never prosecuted for sodomy, Hardwick challenged the Georgia law on grounds that it violated his right to privacy.

Excerpted from the U.S. Supreme Court Decision on the Georgia Sodomy Law, June 30, 1986.

Four justices dissented from the majority opinion ruling that homosexual conduct is not protected by the constitution. Justice Blackmun and Justice Stevens both wrote strongly worded dissenting opinions that pleaded for expanding the zone of privacy to include all forms of human sexuality, traditional or not, as long as the parties are consenting adults. The following reading presents excerpts from the opinions of Justice White and Justice Stevens.

Points to Consider

1. According to Justice White, what issue is being decided?
2. What issues are not addressed?
3. Why do laws against sodomy have ancient roots?
4. How many states have sodomy laws?
5. For what reasons does Justice Stevens dissent from Justice White's majority opinion?

Justice White, *delivered the opinion of the Court.*

In August 1982, respondent was charged with violating the Georgia statute criminalizing sodomy by committing that act with another adult male in the bedroom of respondent's home. . . .

Respondent then brought suit in the Federal District Court, challenging the constitutionality of the statute insofar as it criminalized consensual sodomy. He asserted that he was a practicing homosexual, that the Georgia sodomy statute, as administered by the defendants, placed him in imminent danger of arrest, and that the statute for several reasons violates the Federal Constitution. . . .

The Issue

This case does not require a judgment on whether laws against sodomy between consenting adults in general, or between homosexuals in particular, are wise or desirable. It raises no question about the right or propriety of state legislative decisions to repeal their laws that criminalize homosexual sodomy, or of state court decisions invalidating those laws on state constitutional grounds. The issue presented is whether the Federal Constitution confers a fundamental right upon homosexuals to engage in sodomy and hence invalidates the laws of the many States that still make such conduct illegal and have done so for a very long time. The case also calls for some judgment about the limits of the Court's role in carrying out its constitutional mandate.

We first register our disagreement with the Court of Appeals and with respondent that the Court's prior cases have construed the Constitution to confer a right of privacy that extends to homosexual sodomy and for all intents and purposes have decided this case. . . .

Accepting the decisions in these cases, we think it evident that none of the rights announced in those cases bears any resemblance to the claimed constitutional right of homosexuals to engage in acts of sodomy that is asserted in this case. No connection between family, marriage, or procreation on the one hand and homosexual activity on the other has been demonstrated, either by the Court of Appeals or by respondent. Moreover, any claim that these cases nevertheless stand for the proposition that any kind of private sexual conduct between consenting adults is constitutionally insulated from state proscription is unsupportable. Indeed, the Court's opinion in *Carey* twice asserted that the privacy right, which the *Griswold* line of cases found to be one of the protections provided by the Due Process Clause, did not reach so far. 431 U.S., at 688, n. 5, 694, n. 17.

Precedent aside, however, respondent would have us announce, as the Court of Appeals did, a fundamental right to engage in homosexual sodomy. This we are quite unwilling to do. . . .

Proscriptions against that conduct have ancient roots. . . .Sodomy was a criminal offense at common law and was forbidden by the laws of the original thirteen States when they ratified the Bill of Rights. In 1868, when the Fourteenth Amendment was ratified, all but 5 of the 37 States in the Union had criminal sodomy laws. In fact, until 1961, all 50 States outlawed sodomy, and today, 24 States and the District of Columbia continue to provide criminal penalties for sodomy performed in private and between consenting adults. . . .Against this background, to claim that a right to engage in such conduct is "deeply rooted in this Nation's history and tradition" or "implicit in the concept of ordered liberty" is, at best, facetious.

Nor are we inclined to take a more expansive view of our

authority to discover new fundamental rights imbedded in the Due Process Clause. The Court is most vulnerable and comes nearest to illegitimacy when it deals with judge-made constitutional law having little or no cognizable roots in the language or design of the Constitution. . . .

There should be, therefore, great resistance to expand the substantive reach particulary if it requires redefining the category of rights deemed to be fundamental. Otherwise, the Judiciary necessarily takes to itself further authority to govern the country without express constitutional authority. The claimed right pressed on us today falls far short of over-coming this resistance.

Privacy of the Home

Respondent, however, asserts that the result should be different where the homosexual conduct occurs in the privacy of the home. He relies on *Stanley v. Georgia,* 394 U.S. 557 (1969), where the Court held that the First Amendment prevents conviction for possessing and reading obscene material in the privacy of his home: "If the First Amendment means anything, it means that a State has no business telling a man, sitting alone in his house, what books he may read or what films he may watch."

Stanley did protect conduct that would not have been protected outside the home, and it partially prevented the enforcement of state obscenity laws; but the decision was firmly grounded in the First Amendment. The right pressed upon us here has no similar support in the text of the Constitution, and it does not qualify for recognition under the prevailing principles for construing the Fourteenth Amendment. Its limits are also difficult to discern. Plainly enough, otherwise illegal conduct is not always immunized whenever it occurs in the home. Victimless crimes, such as the possession and use of illegal drugs do not escape the law where they are committed at home. *Stanley* itself recognized that its holding offered no protection for the possession in the home of drugs, firearms, or stolen goods. And if respondent's submission is limited to the voluntary sexual conduct between consenting adults, it would be difficult, except by fiat, to limit the claimed right to homosexual conduct while leaving exposed to prosecution adultery, incest, and other

The Green Light

In upholding the Georgia law, the Court has given a green light to conservative and religious activists around the country to seek legislation protecting their families and communities by restricting the activities of homosexuals. Indeed, leading homosexual leaders fear the decision will blunt or end the homosexual drive for certain job and child custody rights, as well as other goals.

Human Events, *July 12, 1986*

sexual crimes even though they are committed in the home. We are unwilling to start down that road.

Even if the conduct at issue here is not a fundamental right, respondent asserts that there must be a rational basis for the law and that there is none in this case other than the presumed belief of a majority of the electorate in Georgia that homosexual sodomy is immoral and unacceptable. This is said to be an inadequate rationale to support the law. The law, however, is constantly based on notions of morality, and if all laws representing essentially moral choices are to be invalidated under the Due Process Clause, the courts will be very busy indeed. Even respondent makes no such claim, but insists that majority sentiments about the morality of homosexuality should be declared inadequate. We do not agree, and are unpersuaded that the sodomy laws of some 25 States should be invalidated on this basis.

Accordingly, the judgment of the Court of Appeals is *reversed.*

Justice Stevens, *with whom Justice Brennan and Justice Marshall join, dissenting.*

Like the statute that is challenged in this case, the rationale of the Court's opinion applies equally to the prohibited conduct regardless of whether the parties who engage in it are married or unmarried, or are of the same or different sexes. Sodomy was condemned as an odious and sinful type of behavior during the formative period of the common law.

That condemnation was equally damning for heterosexual and homosexual sodomy. Moreover, it provided no special exemption for married couples. The license to cohabit and to produce legitimate offspring simply did not include any permission to engage in sexual conduct that was considered a "crime against nature."

The history of the Georgia statute before us clearly reveals this traditional prohibition of heterosexual, as well as homosexual, sodomy. Indeed, at one point in the 20th century, Georgia's law was construed to permit certain sexual conduct between homosexual women even though such conduct was prohibited between heterosexuals. . . .

Tradition and Liberty

First, the fact that the governing majority in a State has traditionally viewed a particular practice as immoral is not a sufficient reason for upholding a law prohibiting the practice; neither history nor tradition could save a law prohibiting miscegenation from constitutional attack. Second, individual decisions by married persons, concerning the intimacies of their physical relationship, even when not intended to produce offspring, are a form of "liberty" protected by the Due Process Clause of the Fourteenth Amendment. *Griswold v. Connecticut,* 381 U.S. 479 (1965). Moreover, this protection extends to intimate choices by unmarried as well as married persons. *Carey v. Population Services International.* 431 U.S. 678 (1977); *Eisenstadt v. Baird,* 405 U.S. 438 (1972). . . .

Society has every right to encourage its individual members to follow particular traditions in expressing affection for one another and in gratifying their personal desires. It, of course, may prohibit an individual from imposing his will on another to satisfy his own selfish interests. It also may prevent an individual from interfering with, or violating, a legally sanctioned and protected relationship, such as marriage. And it may explain the relative advantages and disadvantages of different forms of intimate expression. But when individual married couples are isolated from observation by others, the way in which they voluntarily choose to conduct their intimate relations is a matter for them—not the State—to decide. The essential "liberty" that animated the development of the law in cases like *Griswold, Eisenstadt,* and *Carey* surely embraces the right to engage in nonreproductive, sexual conduct that others may consider offensive or immoral.

Paradoxical as it may seem, our prior cases thus establish that a State may not prohibit sodomy within "the sacred precincts of marital bedrooms," *Griswold,* 381 U.S. at 485, or, indeed, between unmarried heterosexual adults. *Eisenstadt,* 405 U.S., at 453. In all events, it is perfectly clear that the State of Georgia may not totally prohibit the conduct proscribed by §16-6-2 of the Georgia Criminal Code.

The Georgia Law

If the Georgia statute cannot be enforced as it is written—if the conduct it seeks to prohibit is a protected form of liberty for the vast majority of Georgia's citizens—the State must assume the burden of justifying a selective application of its law. Either the persons to whom Georgia seeks to apply its statute do not have the same interest in "liberty" that others have, or there must be a reason why the State may be permitted to apply a generally applicable law to certain persons that it does not apply to others. . . .

Although the meaning of the principle that "all men are created equal" is not always clear, it surely must mean that every free citizen has the same interest in "liberty" that the members of the majority share. From the standpoint of the individual, the homosexual and the heterosexual have the same interest in deciding how he will live his own life, and,

153

more narrowly, how he will conduct himself in his personal and voluntary associations with his companions. State intrusion into the private conduct of either is equally burdensome.

The second possibility is similarly unacceptable. A policy of selective application must be supported by a neutral and legitimate interest—something more substantial than a habitual dislike for, or ignorance about, the disfavored group. Neither the State nor the Court has identified any such interest in this case. The Court has posited as a justification for the Georgia statute "the presumed belief of a majority of the electorate in Georgia that homosexual sodomy is immoral and unacceptable." But the Georgia electorate has expressed no such belief—instead, its representatives enacted a law that presumably reflects the belief that *all sodomy* is immoral and unacceptable. Unless the Court is prepared to conclude that such a law is constitutional, it may not rely on the work product of the Georgia Legislature to support its holding. For the Georgia statute does not single out homosexuals as a separate class meriting special disfavored treatment.

Nor, indeed, does the Georgia prosecutor even believe that all homosexuals who violate this statute should be punished. This conclusion is evident from the fact that the respondent in this very case has formally acknowledged in his complaint and in court that he has engaged, and intends to continue to engage, in the prohibited conduct, yet the State has elected not to process criminal charges against him. As Justice Powell points out, moreover, Georgia's prohibition on private, consensual sodomy has not been enforced for decades." The record of nonenforcement, in this case and in the last several decades, belies the Attorney General's representations about the importance of the State's selective application of its generally applicable law.

Both the Georgia statute and the Georgia prosecutor thus completely fail to provide the Court with any support for the conclusion that homosexual sodomy is considered unacceptable conduct in that State, and that the burden of justifying a selective application of the generally applicable law has been met.

EXAMINING
COUNTERPOINTS

This activity may be used as an individualized study guide for students in libraries and resource centers or as a discussion catalyst in small group and classroom discussions.

Guidelines

•Social issues are usually complex, but often problems become oversimplified in political debates and discussion. Usually a polarized version of social conflict does not adequately represent the diversity of views that surround social conflicts.
•Examine the overview of Proposition 64 (The California AIDS Initiative) and the counterpoints that follow. Then think about and discuss the merits of Proposition 64.

Overview: Proposition 64 - July, 1986

This measure declares that AIDS and the "condition of being a carrier" of the virus that causes AIDS are communicable diseases. The measure also requires the State Department of Health Services to add these conditions to the list of diseases that must be reported. Because AIDS cases are already being reported, the measure would require the reporting of those who are "carriers of the AIDS virus." Currently, no test to make this determination is readily available.

The measure also states that the Department of Health Services and all health officers "shall fulfill all of the duties and obligations specified" under the applicable laws "in a manner consistent with the intent of this act." Although the meaning of this language could be subject to two different interpretations, it most likely means that the laws and regulations which currently apply to other communicable diseases shall also apply to AIDS and the "condition of being a carrier" of the AIDS virus. Thus, health officers would continue to exercise their discretion in taking actions necessary to control this disease. Based on existing medical knowledge and health department practices, few, if any, AIDS patients and carriers of the AIDS virus would be placed in isolation or under quarantine. Similarly, few, if any, persons would be excluded from schools or food handling jobs. If, however, the language is interpreted as placing new requirements on health officers, it could result in new actions such as expanding testing programs for the AIDS virus, imposing isolation or quarantine of persons who have the disease, and excluding persons infected with the AIDS virus from schools and food handling positions.

The fiscal effect of this measure could vary greatly, depending on how it would be interpreted by state and local health officers and the courts. If existing discretionary communicable disease controls were applied to the AIDS disease, there would be no substantial net change in state and local costs as a direct result of this measure. Thus, the primary effect of this measure would be to require the reporting of persons who are carriers of the virus which causes AIDS. Very few cases would be reported because no test to confirm that a person carries the virus is readily available. If such a test becomes widely available in the future, more cases would be reported.

The fiscal impact could be very substantial if the measure were interpreted to require changes in AIDS control measures by state and local health officers, either voluntarily or as a result of a change in medical knowledge on how the disease is spread, or as a result of court decisions which mandate certain control measures. Ultimately, the fiscal impact would depend on the level of activity that state and local health officers might undertake with respect to: (1) identifying, isolating and quarantining persons infected with the virus, or having the disease, and (2) excluding those persons from schools or food handling positions. The cost of implementing these actions could range from millions of dollars to hundreds of millions of dollars per year.

In summary, the net fiscal impact of this measure is unknown—and could vary greatly, depending on what actions are taken by health officers and the courts to implement this measure.

The Point: Argument in Favor of Proposition 64

Proposition 64 extends existing public health codes for communicable diseases, to AIDS and AIDS virus carriers. This means that the same public health codes that already protect you and your family from other dangerous diseases, will also protect you from AIDS. Proposition 64 will keep AIDS out of our schools, out of commercial food establishments, and will give health officials the power to test and quarantine where needed. These measures are not new; they are the same health measures applied, by law, every day, to every other dangerous contagious disease.

Today AIDS is out of control. There are at least 300,000 AIDS carriers in California and the number of cases of this highly contagious disease is doubling every 6 to 12 months. The number of "unexplained" AIDS cases—cases not in "high-risk" groups, such as homosexuals and intravenous drug-users—continues to grow at alarming rates. Indeed, the majority of cases worldwide fall into no identifiable "risk-group" whatsoever. The AIDS virus has been found living in many bodily fluids, including blood, saliva, respiratory fluids, sweat, and tears, and it can survive upwards of seven days outside the body. There presently exists no cure for the sick, and no vaccination for the healthy. It is 100% lethal.

AIDS is the gravest public health threat our nation has ever faced. The existing law of California clearly states that certain proven public health measures must be taken to protect the public from any communicable disease, and no competent medical professional denies that AIDS is "communicable." Despite these facts, politicians and special interest groups have circumvented the public health laws. For the first time in our history, a deadly disease is being treated as a "civil rights"issue, rather than as a public health issue.

The medical facts are clear. The law is clear. Common sense agrees. You and your family have the right to be protected from all contagious diseases, including AIDS—the deadliest of them all. If you agree, vote YES on Proposition 64.

KHUSHRO GHANDHI
California Director,
National Democratic Policy Committee (NDPC),
and Member-elect, Los Angeles County
Democratic Party Central Committee

JOHN GRAUERHOLZ, M.D., FCAP (Fellow, College of American Pathologists)

The Counterpoint: Argument Against Proposition 64

Proposition 64 must be defeated for the Safety and Public Health of all Californians. It is an irrational, inappropriate and misguided approach to a serious public health problem. The proponents of this measure are followers of extremist Lyndon LaRouche. They want to create an atmosphere of fear, misunderstanding, inadequate health care and panic. In fact, the acronym of their campaign committee is PANIC.

Public health decisions must be left in the hands of the medical profession and public health officials or we will endanger the lives of Californians. The California Medical Association and County Public Health officials recognize the danger of allowing political extremists to dictate state public health and medical policy.

This type of repressive and discriminatory action forced upon Californians by followers of Lyndon LaRouche will not serve to limit the problem, but rather could prolong the spread of this terrible disease. The fear of quarantine or other discriminatory measures, including loss of jobs, will make people reluctant to be tested. Fearing social isolation, individuals at risk will avoid early medical intervention, or even infection testing, driving AIDS underground.

Enforcement of this measure could cost the taxpayers billions of dollars to quarantine and isolate AIDS carriers and could require public health officials to do so. Quarantine would serve no medical purpose because there are no documented cases of AIDS ever being transmitted by casual contact.

158

Californians from all walks of life know they must unite to end this dreadful epidemic. Californians can be proud that doctors and public health officials have acted in a professional, rational and responsible manner to protect the health of Californians and have taken all appropriate precautions as they are needed. This kind of initiative can only divide, create panic and force thousands not to get tested or treated because of fear.

Join us, the Los Angeles Times, The Los Angeles Herald Examiner, San Francisco Examiner, The California Medical Association, and many others in opposing the extremes of followers of Lyndon LaRouche. Vote NO on Proposition 64!

GLADDEN V. ELLIOT, M.D.
President
California Medical Association

ED ZSCHAU
Member of Congress

ALAN CRANSTON
United States Senator

BIBLIOGRAPHY

Research and Epidemiology
of AIDS

"Acquired immune deficiency syndrome." **Time,** v. 122, July 4, 1983: 50-58. Contents.–Hunting for the hidden killers, by W. Isaacson.–The real epidemic: fear and despair, by J. Leo.

"Acquired Immunodeficiency Syndrome in Infants." **New England Journal of Medicine,** v. 310, Jan. 12, 1984: 76-81. "This report describes a series of 14 infants, predominantly American-born Haitian infants with characteristics of a profound cellular immune deficiency and multiple infections, who were seen in Miami over a 32-month period from November 1980 through June 1983."

"The Acquired Immunodeficiency Syndrome." **JAMA** [Journal of the American Medical Association], v. 252, Oct. 19, 1984: 2037-2043. Reviews the development of AIDS as a major public health problem in the U.S. Describes the etiology, problems of diagnosis, patient evaluation and treatment, means of transmission, and prevention of the disease.

AIDS: Chapter One. Boston, WGBH Transcripts, 1985. 23 p. (NOVA no. 1205) Transcript of NOVA television program examines Acquired Immune Deficiency Syndrome and the works of epidemiologists who are studying the disease.

Altman, Lawrence K. "AIDS in Africa: A Pattern of Mystery." **New York Times,** Nov. 8, 1985: A1, A8. Emphasizes that the epidemiology of AIDS is very different in Africa than elsewhere. Researchers have found that AIDS is spreading by conventional sexual intercourse among heterosexuals and is striking nearly as many women as men, with transmission to newborn infants a growing problem.

DeCock, Kevin M. "AIDS: An Old Disease from Africa?" **British Medical Journal,** v. 289, Aug. 4, 1984: 306-308. "Proposes that the infectious agent causing AIDS, whatever its nature, is endemic and unrecognized in parts of sub-Saharan Africa, from where it recently disseminated into external populations. No other explanation unifies the confusing observations on the syndrome."

DePalma, Anthony. "The Children's Crusader." **New Jersey Monthly,** v. 11, Feb. 1986: 49-52, 54-55, 140. Profiles Dr. James Oleske, an immunologist at Children's Hospital in Newark, who was one of the first physicians in the country to detect AIDS in children.

The Epidemiology of AIDS: Current Status and Future Prospects. **Science,** v. 229, Sept. 27, 1985: 1352-1357. Illustrates the rate at which AIDS has spread within the United States and other countries. Describes modes of transmission for the disease.

Gelman, David. "AIDS." **Newsweek,** v. 106, Aug. 12, 1985: 20-24, 26-29. Points out that AIDS is not restricted to homosexuals and warns that AIDS could "become one of those infectious diseases that change history."

"The Incidence Rate of Acquired Immunodeficiency Syndrome in Selected Populations." **JAMA** [Journal of the American Medical Association], v. 253, Jan. 11, 1985: 215-220.

"Intra-blood-brain-barrier Synthesis of HTLV-III-specific IgG in Patients with Neurologic Symptoms Associated with AIDS or AIDS-related Complex." **New England Journal of Medicine,** v. 313, Dec. 12, 1985: 1498-1504. Notes that "central nervous system dysfunction [such as dementia] occurs frequently in patients with AIDS."

"Lack of Transmission of HTLV-III/LAV Infection to Household Contacts of Patients with AIDS or AIDS-related Complex with Oral Candidiasis."**New England Journal of Medicine,** v. 314, Feb. 6, 1986: 344-349. In this study, 101 nonsexual household contacts of 39 patients with AIDS or AIDS-related complex were interviewed and tested for the AIDS virus. These contacts had shared household items and facilities and had close personal interaction with the patients for a median of 22 months. Only one contact, a five year old child, had evidence of infection, which was probably acquired perinatally.

Langone, John. "AIDS." **Discover,** v. 6, Dec. 1985: 28-33, 36, 38-42, 44-45, 48-50, 52-53. Notes that the AIDS virus does not spread easily, its targets are highly selected and predictable.

Laurence, Jeffrey. "The Immune System in AIDS." **Scientific American,** v. 253, Dec. 1985: 84-93. "The AIDS virus alters the growth and function of T4 lymphocytes, a class of white cells that is crucial to the immune system. New knowledge of how the virus does so may lead to treatments and perhaps a vaccine."

Marwick, Charles. "AIDS-associated Virus Yields Data to Intensifying Scientific Study." **JAMA** [Journal of the American Medical Association], v. 254, Nov. 22-29, 1985: 2865-2870. Contends that the AIDS virus is probably not very contagious, even though it is possible to get the disease "from a single sexual encounter with someone who has AIDS or by receiving a single unit of blood that has the virus in it."

Meyer, Harry M. "Food and Drug Administration Responses to the Challenges of AIDS." **Public Health Reports,** v. 98, July-Aug. 1983: 320-323. "Research and policy actions that FDA has initiated have been designed to ensure as fully as possible the safety and effectiveness of regulated products that are relevant to AIDS and to apply new technology to this important public health problem."

Norman, Colin. "The War on AIDS." **Science,** v. 230, Oct. 25, 1985: 418-419; Nov. 1: 518-521; Nov. 8: 640-642; Nov. 29: 1018-1021; Dec. 6: 1140-1142; Dec. 20: 1355-1358. Contents.–Congress readies AIDS funding transfusion.–AIDS virology: a battle on many fronts.–Patent dispute divides AIDS researchers.–AIDS trends: projections from limited data.–Politics and science clash on African AIDS.–AIDS therapy: new use for clinical trials.

"Patients at Risk for AIDS–related Opportunistic Infections." **New England Journal of Medicine,** v. 313, Dec. 12, 1985: 1504-1510.

Peterman, Thomas A., Peter D. Drotman, and James W. Curran. "Epidemiology of the Acquired Immunodeficiency Syndrome (AIDS)." **Epidemologic Reviews,** v. 7, 1985: 1-21. Presents the etiology of AIDS and describes how the disease has spread. Contains an extensive bibliography.

Randal, Judith. "Too Little Aid for AIDS." **Technology Review,** v. 87, Aug.-Sept. 1984: 10, 12-13, 79. Contends that the Reagan Administration has not really given much assistance to the Centers for Disease Control and NIH for fighting AIDS. Reveals that CDC has had to take money from other programs in order to fund AIDS research.

Redfield, Robert R. "Heterosexually Acquired HTLV-III/LAV Disease (AIDS-related complex and AIDS): Epidemiologic Evidence for Female-to-Male Transmission." **JAMA** [Journal of the American Medical Association], v. 254, Oct. 18, 1985: 2094-2096. "Provides further epidemiologic evidence to support the occurrence of bidirectional heterosexual transmission (both male to female and female to male) of AIDS.

Review of the Public Health Service's Response to AIDS. Washington, Office of Technology Assessment, for sale by the Supt. of Docs., G.P.O., 1985. 158 p. "OTA-TM-H-24"

"Screening Test for HTLV-III (AIDS agent) Antibodies: Specificity, Sensitivity, and Applications." **JAMA** [Journal of the American Medical Association], v. 253, Jan. 11, 1985: 221-225.

Taylor, Nick. "Racing Against the AIDS Clock: The Challenge at CDC." **Atlanta Magazine,** v. 23, Jan. 1984: 38-41. Profiles the AIDS Task Force at the Centers for Disease Control.

"Transfusion-associated Acquired Immunodeficiency Syndrome in the United States." **JAMA** [Journal of the American Medical Association], v. 254, Nov. 22-29, 1985: 2913-2917. "The risk of developing AIDS after a blood transfusion has been low and will be lowered further by using both self-deferral and antibody screening."

"U.S., French Studies Link Leukemia Virus to AIDS." **Hospital Practice,** v. 18, July 1983: 33, 37-38, 40-41. "Four studies in the United States and France suggest that infection with a recently discovered human retrovirus–human T-cell leukemia virus (HTLV)–may be involved in acquired immune deficiency syndrome (AIDS)."

Wallis, Claudia. "AIDS: a Growing Threat." **Time,** v. 126, Aug. 12, 1985: 40-47. Describes how AIDS attacks the immune system and how AIDS victims succumb to opportunistic infections.

Weber, Jonathan. "AIDS: The Virus Is Not Immune." **New Scientist,** v. 109: Jan. 2, 1986: 37-39. "Although we still have no specific cure for the disease doctors have identified the most promising strategies for combating the AIDS virus and its devastating effects on the human body."

Spread of AIDS

Anderson, Gary R. "Children and AIDS: implications for child welfare." **Child Welfare,** v. 63, Jan.-Feb. 1984: 62-73. Discusses the history and background of AIDS and its symptoms, means of transmission and methods of treatment in adults and children.

Baum, Rudy M. "AIDS Epidemic Continues, Moving Beyond High-risk Groups." **Chemical & Engineering News,** v. 63, Apr. 1, 1985: 19-22, 25-26. "Despite the significant scientific advances, very little is known about how the virus attacks its victims' immune systems. Development of a vaccine against the virus, althought the goal of many researchers, is not yet on the horizon and may not be possible."

Gelman, David. "AIDS." **Newsweek,** v. 106, Aug. 12, 1985: 20-24, 26-29. Tracks the spread of acquired immune deficiency syndrome. Points out that AIDS is not restricted to homosexuals and warns that AIDS could "become one of those infectious diseases that change history." Contains a poll showing increasing concern about AIDS.

Ginzburg, Harold M. "Intravenous Drug Users and the Acquired Immune Deficiency Syndrome." **Public Health Reports,** v. 99, Mar.-Apr. 1984: 206-212. "Focuses on drug users who may be most at risk for AIDS, the concerns of drug users about AIDS, and the concerns of their treatment service providers."

"Immunodeficiency in Female Sexual partners of Men with the Acquired Immuno-Deficiency Syndrome." **New England Journal of Medicine,** v. 30, May 19, 1983: 1181-1184. Studies seven female sexual partners of male patients with AIDS. "Findings suggest that AIDS may be transmitted between heterosexual men and women."

"The Incidence Rate of Acquired Immunodeficiency Syndrome in Selected Populations." **JAMA** [Journal of the American Medical Association], v. 253, Jan. 11, 1985: 215-220. Reports results of a statistical study of incidence of AIDS in single men, IV drug users, Haitians living in the U.S., persons with hemophilia, and recipients of blood transfusions.

Ioachim, Harry L., Chester W. Lerner and Michael L. Tapper. "Lymphadenopathies in Homosexual Men: Relationships with the Acquired Immune Deficiency Syndrome." **JAMA** [Journal of the American Medical Association], v. 250, Sept. 9, 1983: 1306-1309. Evaluates persistent lymphadenopathies in homosexual men as precursors of acquired immune deficiency syndrome.

Wallis, Claudia. "AIDS: a Growing Threat." **Time,** v. 126, Aug. 12, 1985: 40-47.

Blood Supply

"Acquired Immunodeficiency Syndrome (AIDS) Associated with Transfusions." **New England Journal of Medicine,** v. 310, Jan. 12, 1984: 69-75. This "description of 18 adults without other risk factors in whom AIDS developed after transfusion indicates that other blood components may transmit AIDS."

Blood Policy & Technology. Washington, Office of Technology Assessment, for sale by the Supt. of Docs., G.P.O., 1985. 240 p. "Transfusion-related cases of acquired immunodeficiency syndrome (AIDS) have threatened the safety of the blood supply and the equanimity that has been the foundation of the voluntary blood donor system."

Cooper, Ann. The High-stakes Race is On to Develop Blood Test to Detect AIDS Virus. **National Journal,** v. 16, Aug. 4, 1984: 1470-1472. "Blood banks and some doctors fear the test being developed by private firms will not be reliable, and gay rights groups worry about discriminatory uses of test results."

Eckert, Ross D., and Edward L. Wallace. **Securing a Safer Blood Supply: Two Views.** Washington, American Enterprise Institute for Public Policy Research, 1985. 153 p. (AEI studies, no. 416) The authors present opposing views on how the Nation's blood services system should be structured to insure a safe supply of blood.

Screening Test for HTLV-III (AIDS agent) Antibodies: Specificity, Sensitivity, and Applications. **JAMA** [Journal of the American Medical Association], v. 253, Jan. 11, 1985: 221-225. Claims development of a test for HTLV-III antibodies which "will be a useful screening test among blood donors and populations at risk for AIDS, will aid in the diagnosis of suspected AIDS, and will help in defining the spectrum of diseases that are etiologicially related to HTLV-III."

Ethical and Legal Issues

"AIDS." **Issues in Science and Technology,** v. 2, winter 1986: 39-73. Contents.–The AIDS epidemic: an overview of the science, by J. Osborn.–AIDS and ethics, by A. Jonsen, M. Cooke, and B. Koenig.–AIDS: allocating resources for research and patient care, by P. Lee.

AIDS: The Merging Ethical Dilemmas. **Hastings Center Report,** Aug. 1985, suppl.: 1-32. Partial contents.–AIDS: the challenge to science and medicine, by M. Krim.–Screening blood: public health and medical uncertainty, by C. Levine and R. Bayer.–AIDS and the threat to public health, by M. Silverman and D. Silverman.–AIDS: public policy and biomedical research, by S. Panem.

AIDS: What Is To Be Done? **Harper's Magazine,** v. 271, Oct. 1985: 39-52. Presents a transcript of a discussion among a group of public health officials, physicians, scientists, and medical historians on what can be done to contain AIDS.

Blau, Robert, "Blood Feud." **Chicago Tribune Magazine,** Dec. 15, 1985: 10-12, 15-16, 18, 20, 29. The use of the test ELISA (energy-linked immunosorbent assay) to screen blood for the HTLV-III virus has given rise to fears the test may be misused.

Cecere, Michael S. "AIDS Presents Many Legal Issues for Workplace." **Legal Times,** v. 8, Dec. 2, 1985: 10, 13-14. Concludes that "AIDS is a protected handicap or disability under federal and state fair employment practice laws. As such, it must be treated like any other handicap or disability."

Collier, Stephen. "Preventing the Spread of AIDS by Restricting Sexual Conduct in Gay Bathhouses: A Constitutional Analysis." **Golden Gate University Law Review,** v. 15, summer 1985: 301-330.

Tarr, Amy. "AIDS: The Legal Issues Widen." **National Law Journal,** v. 8, Nov. 25, 1985: 1, 28-29. "The boundaries of the AIDS legal crisis are being expanded as insurers look for ways to contain claims; employers decide how to deal with workers who have it or have been exposed to it; municipalities search for ways to control and monitor activities believed to contribute to the spread of the disease; and public schools deal with students who have AIDS."

Social and Political Issues

The AIDS Epidemic: A Victim Shares His Story." **Nuestro,** v. 9, Aug. 1985: 22-27. Fourteen percent of AIDS victims are Latinos, yet Latinos only comprise seven percent of the U.S. population.

AIDS Legal Guide: A Professional Resource on AIDS-related Issues and Discrimination. New York, Lambda Legal Defense and Education Fund, 1984. 1 v. (ca. 100 p.) Emphasizes New York State and City law and practices.

"AIDS: Special Report." **Health Magazine** [Washington Post], Sept. 4, 1985: 1-22. In this special report are articles on the AIDS virus, the treatment of the disease, interviews with AIDS patients and medical personnel working with them. A Washington Post poll on AIDS is included.

Black, David. "The Plague Years." **Rolling Stone,** no. 444, Mar. 28, 1985: 48-50, 52, 54, 114, 117, 119-125; no. 446, Apr. 25: 35-36, 39, 41, 43-45, 56-62. In this two part series the author recounts the medical story on the search for a cure for AIDS and examines society's reactions to the disease and homosexuals.

Changing Gay Lifestyles. **Advocate,** no. 379, Oct. 27, 1983: 22-35. Contents.--AIDS and the mind: psychological aspects of a mysterious disease, by N. Fain.–AIDS and moral issues: will sexual liberation survive, by T. Johnson.--An AIDS journal: Mark Feldman's personal battle, by M. Helquist.

Collier, Peter and David Horowitz. "White Wash." **California Magazine,** v. 8, July 1983: 52-57. San Francisco's gay leaders, worried about the image of their community, have obsured the fact that life-style may be an important factor in the spread of the acquired immune deficiency syndrome.

"Gay America in Transition." **Newsweek,** v. 102, Aug. 8, 1983: 30-36, 39-40. Assesses the effect on the gay community of the AIDS epidemic.

Ismach, Judy M. "AIDS: Can the Nation Cope?" **Medical World News,** v. 26, Aug. 26, 1985: 46-48, 51, 54, 59-62, 68, 70-71. Looks at the staggering potential human toll and economic burden on the country's health care system due to AIDS.

Leishman, Katie. "A Crisis in Public Health." **Atlantic Monthly,** v. 256, Oct. 1985: 18, 20-24, 26, 28-31, 34-35, 38, 40-41. Looks at efforts in San Francisco to provide health care to AIDS victims and the city's attempts to educate the public about the disease.

Martin, Thad. "AIDS: Is It a Major Threat to Blacks?" **Ebony,** v. 40, Oct. 1985: 91-92, 96. Of the more than 12,000 reported AIDS cases, 25 percent of the victims are blacks.

McKusick, Leon, William Horstman, and Thomas J. Coates. "AIDS and Sexual Behavior Reported by Gay Men in San Francisco." **American Journal of Public Health,** v. 75, May 1985: 493-496. Tries "to determine whether gay men's sexual behavior had changed since the onset of AIDS in response to the crisis, and to understand better the factors influencing sexual behavior so that future health education programs could be designed accordingly."

Pressman, Steven. "The Gay Community Struggles to Fashion an Effective Lobby." **Congressional Quarterly Weekly Report,** v. 41, Dec. 3, 1983: 2543-2547. "Concerned about the AIDS crisis, gay civil rights and other issues, America's homosexuals are trying to transform a fledgling political movement into a national lobbying force."

Sager, Mike. "The New Scarlet Letter: AIDS." **Washingtonian,** v. 21, Jan. 1986: 104-107, 156-157. Claims that AIDS is not just a medical story. Illustrates how the straight community is using AIDS as a mask for its feelings about homosexuals.

Streitmatter, Rodger. "AIDS: 'It's Just a Matter of Time.' " **Quill,** v. l72, May 1984: 22-27. The author conducted a survey of network news, three major news magazines, six major dailies, and mid-sized TV stations and newspapers from around the U.S. and concludes that the AIDS story was "treated sensationally and irresponsibly by most news media."

Talbot, David, and Larry Bush. "At Risk." **Mother Jones,** v. 10, Apr. 1985: 28-37. Criticizes the Reagan administration's efforts to combat

AIDS. Claims that delays due to inadequate funding may have hurt research efforts.

Thompson, Roger. AIDS: Spreading Mystery Disease. [Washington, Congressional Quarterly] 1985. 599-615 p. (Editorial research reports, 1985, v. 2, no. 6) Contents.–Protecting the public.–Coping with epidemics.–Impact on society.

Waldman, Steven. The Other AIDS Crisis: Who Pays for the Treatment? **Washington Monthly,** v. 17, Jan. 1986: 25-31. Asserts that "the Reagan administration has sponsored research and public education but has generally avoided the issue of who is going to pay for AIDS treatment. Instead, the administration has casually assumed that the private sector, states, and cities, will come to the rescue." Reports that insurance companies are trying to exclude homosexuals.

National AIDS Related Organizations And Information

American Association of Physicians for Human Rights
1050 West Pacific Coast Highway
Harbor City, CA 90701
(213) 584-0491

American Association of Physicians for Human Rights
P.O. Box 143266
San Francisco, CA 94114
(415) 558-9393

American Psychological Association
1200 17th Street, N.W.
Washington, DC 20036
(202) 955-7600

Gay Rights National Lobby/AIDS Project
P.O. Box 1892
Washington, DC 20013
(202) 546-1801

National AIDS/Pre-AIDS Epidemiological Network
2676 North Halsted Street
Chicago, IL 60614
(312) 943-6600 x424, x389

National Association for Lesbian and Gay Gerontology
271 La Casa Avenue
San Mateo, CA 94403
(415) 349-4537

National Coalition of Gay STD Services
P.O. Box 239
Milwaukee, WI 53201-0239
(414) 277-7671

National Gay Health Coalition
206 North 35th Street
Philadelphia, PA 19143
(215) 386-5327

National Gay/Lesbian Health Education Foundation
P.O. Box 784
New York, NY 10036
(212) 563-6313

National Gay Task Force (NGTF)
80 Fifth Avenue
New York, NY 10011
(212) 741-5800

National Gay Rights Advocates (NGRA)
540 Castro Street
San Francisco, CA 94114
(415) 863-3624

Association of Lesbian and Gay Social Workers
1527 Spruce Street, #33
Philadelphia, PA 19102
(215) 985-1581

**National Federation of Parents
& Friends of Gays**
5715 16th Street, N.W.
Washington, DC 20011
(202) 726-3223

National Gay Health Coalition
506 West 42nd Street, #E5
New York, NY 10036
(212) 563-6313

National Association of Lesbian and Gay Gerontologists
3312 Descano Drive
Los Angeles, CA 90026
(213) 661-3138

Lambda Legal Defense & Education Fund
132 West 43rd Street
New York, NY 10036
(212) 944-9488

American Hospital Association
840 North Lake Shore
Chicago, IL
(312) 280-6000

**AIDS Action Council of the Federation
of AIDS-Related Organizations**
1115½ Independence Avenue, S.E.
Washington, DC 20003
(202) 547-3101

**American Mental Health Counselors
Association - Gay/Lesbian Task Force**
502 East Tam-o-Shanter Drive
Phoenix, AZ 85022

Lutherans Concerned (for gay people)
Box 10461, Fort Dearborn Station,
Chicago, Illinois 60610

AIDS Resource Center
235 West 18th Street
New York, NY 10011
(212) 206-1414

American Foundation for AIDS Research
230 Park Avenue
New York, NY 10017
(212) 949-7410

AID Atlanta
811 Cypress Street
Atlanta, GA 30308
(404) 872-0600

Gay Men's Health Crisis
254 West 18th Street
New York, NY 10011
(212) 807-7035

Women's AIDS Network
707 San Bruno Avenue
San Francisco, CA 94107
(415) 821-7984

National Hemophilia Foundation
19 West 34th Street, #1204
New York, NY 10001
(212) 563-0211

**US Department of Health & Human Services,
Public Health Service**
Washington, DC 20201
(202) 245-6867

Centers for Disease Control/AIDS Activity
1600 Clifton Road, N.E.
Atlanta, GA 30333
(404) 329-3311

**American Public Health Association-
Caucus of Gay Public Health Workers**
506 West 42nd Street, #E5
New York, NY 10036

**American Psychiatric Association-
Gay/Lesbian/Bisexual Caucus**
2001 Union Street, #340
San Francisco, CA 94123
(415) 931-4656

**American Psychological Association-
Committee on Gay Concerns**
4328 18th Street
San Francisco, CA 94114

Gay Nurses Alliance
44 St. Marks Place
New York, NY 10003

Lesbian & Gay People in Medicine
1465 Lee Road, P.O. Box 131
Chantilly, VA 22021
(703) 968-7920

National Caucus of Gay & Lesbian Counselors
P.O. Box 216
Jenkintown, PA 19046

**Federation of Parents & Friends
of Lesbians and Gays**
P.O. Box 24565
Los Angeles, CA 90024
(213) 492-8952

Person With AIDS Organizations

People With AIDS-Atlanta
1235 Monroe Street, #1
Atlanta, GA 30306
(404) 892-8766

People With AIDS-Chicago
3414 N. Halsted Street
Chicago, IL 60657
(312) 327-9564

People With AIDS-Los Angeles
1752 North Fuller
Los Angeles, CA 90046

People With AIDS-New York
444 Hudson, #G27
New York, NY 10011

People With AIDS-Dallas
3409 Oak Lawn, #202
Dallas, TX 75219

People With AIDS-San Francisco
519 Castro Street, #146
San Francisco, CA 94114

Pamphlets And Packets

AIDS Information Packet
Center for Disease Control
1600 Clifton Road Northeast
Atlanta, GA 30333
(404) 329-3311

"A Complete Workshop Outline for Pastoral Care Providers"
AID Atlanta, 811 Cypress Street
Atlanta, GA 30308
(404) 872-0600

"Guidelines on AIDS in the Workplace,"
Department of Health
and Human Services
Office of the Assistant Secretary for Health
Washington, D.C. 20201

"Guidelines: A Hospitalwide Approach to AIDS"
Developed by The American Hospital Association Advisory Committee on Infections within Hospitals, in consultation with the Center for Disease Control.
The American Hospital Association
840 North Lake Shore Drive
Chicago, IL 60611
(312) 280-6000

"An Ounce of Prevention"
AIDS risk reduction guidelines by New York Physicians for
Human Rights, GMHC Inc.
Box 274, 132 West 24th Street
Ney York, NY 10011
(212) 807-6655 (A self-addressed, stamped return envelope)

"Human Sexuality and Sexual Behavior"
ALC statement of comment and counsel, 1980
Augsburg Publishing House,
426 South Fifth Street
Minneapolis, MN 55415

AIDS Telephone Hotlines

National AIDS telephone hotline—1-800/447-2437
Atlanta area: (404) 329-1295
GMHC—Hotline (New York), (212) 807-6655

AIDS Research And Experimental Therapies

Hundreds of drugs have been screened to find substances effective in treating AIDS or AIDS-related conditions, including: 1) antivirals, which may act against the HTLV-III virus; 2) immune modulators, that might bolster the immune system; 3) combinations of therapies; and 4) drugs that might be effective against AIDS-related "opportunistic" infections.

AIDS Vaccine—A vaccine based on the classic polio vaccine has protected monkeys from a deadly AIDS-like virus for more than a year, say researchers at the University of California at Davis. . . ."The (Davis) work is a significant report," said Dr. Jonas Salk, who developed the polio vaccine in 1954 and who now heads the Salk Institute in San Diego. "It lays the foundation for future work on the same lines, mainly that of developing a non-infectious vaccine for AIDS." (Associated Press, September 3, 1986)

New Treatment—University of Minnesota doctors plan to try novel types of white-blood-cell infusions as experimental treatment for 12 AIDS patients and a dozen people with advanced cancer. The technique has been used to turn ordinary white blood cells into roving cancer "killers" at the federal National Cancer Institute in Bethesda, MD. Researchers there reported encouraging early results last month in 11 patients, but cautioned that it's too early to claim long-term success. (Lewis Cope in the *Minneapolis Star and Tribune,* January 18, 1986)

Scientists Grow AIDS Virus—Researchers have successfully grown the virus that causes AIDS in animal cells for the first time, a development they say could lead to finding ways to inhibit reproduction of the deadly organism. . . . The virus reproduced poorly in these cells, especially mouse cells, a fact that could be very useful in future research, said Dr. Jay A. Levy, principal investigator of the study at the university.

173

. . ."If we can learn how mouse cells limit the AIDS virus growth, we may be able to find a way to suppress the virus growth in humans," he said. "The slow growth in animal cells also suggests that the AIDS virus has adapted to humans, and has probably been in the human population for some time." (Associated Press, May 16, 1986)

AIDS in Sperm—Widespread use of fresh sperm for artificial insemination is "clearly hazardous" because of the risk of transmitting AIDS and other diseases, and doctors should impregnate women only with frozen sperm that has been checked for germs, a federal report concludes. The researchers said 80 percent to 90 percent of artificial inseminations in the United States are performed with fresh sperm. Between 6,000 and 10,000 births result from artificial insemination each year. (Associated Press, May 22, 1986)

Killing AIDS Virus—Scientists have learned for the first time how to kill the AIDS virus, independent research teams at Harvard and the National Cancer Institute said Thursday. By removing a key gene from the HTLV-III virus in laboratory experiments, the researchers rendered the virus harmless— an advance that may lead to drugs or a vaccine to combat the deadly disease. *(Los Angeles Times, March 28, 1986)*

Gene-engineered AIDS Vaccine—Two processes describ- ed as "the very first steps" toward a possible AIDS vaccine were announced by genetic engineers Monday at a world AIDS conference. Coupled with the announcements were warnings that a practical vaccine could be a long time com- ing. . . .Genentech, Inc., of San Francisco, and Oncogen of Seattle, working with Transgene of Strasbourg, France, reported successful experiments of genetically engineered products that prevented AIDS in the test tube. *(Minneapolis Star and Tribune, June 7, 1986)*

New Mutant Virus—The National Cancer Institute said researchers have created a nondeadly version of the AIDS virus, raising hopes the mutant can be used to develop a treatment or vaccine. . . .Researchers also are continuing work aimed at developing a vaccine, which probably would contain some form of the AIDS virus. The advantage of basing it instead on the nondeadly mutant would be in putting a layer of safety between the original virus and the person who would be getting the vaccine, she said. (News Services, August 1, 1986)

Scientists Find New AIDS Virus—A government scientist has reported the discovery of an unknown virus among AIDS patients. Other scientists say the finding has opened up wide possibilities that need to be explored in further research. *(New York Times,* August 3, 1986)

New Drug Tests—About 3,000 AIDS patients—out of more than 23,000 who have been afflicted with the disease—are participating in clinical trials at medical centers around the country. Half a dozen drugs are being tested. The federal government recently announced that it would enroll an additional 1,000 patients in new programs within the next six months and release $100 million over the next five years in a further expansion of its involvement in experimental AIDS treatment. *(Los Angeles Times,* August 3, 1986)

New Genetic Trigger—A new genetic trigger has been discovered that is essential for the growth and spread of the AIDS virus, and scientists say it may provide another target for drugs to attack the lethal microbe. The gene, called art, is the seventh AIDS gene discovered as researchers rapidly expand their knowledge of the virus' inner workings. (Associated Press, May 22, 1986)

AIDS And Insects—A leading French scientist has found that many insects in central Africa are infected with the AIDS virus and that such insects may be able to transmit the disease to humans in certain regions. The report drew skepticism from some American AIDS researchers. . . .In Belle Glade, Fla., the town that has the highest per-capita rate of AIDS cases in the United States, Dr. Mark Whiteside has said AIDS virus-carrying mosquitoes may be part of the problem. In February the Centers for Disease Control launched an extensive study in Belle Glade intended in part to explore Whiteside's speculation. (*Los Angeles Times*, August 26, 1986)

Promising New Drug—Federal Health officials are expected to announce today that an experimental AIDS drug has shown such early promise that it should be made more widely available to people suffering from the deadly disease, Department of Health and Human Services sources said. Azidothymidine (AZT) is the first drug shown to have prolonged AIDS patients' survival, although researchers and other health officials stressed that it is neither a cure nor a breakthrough drug, and they are uncertain of its long-term effects.